# Anti-Inflammatory Cookbook for Beginners

## Meal plans to help combat Inflammation

Charles Jefferson

Abel Moore

# Copyright © [2024] by Charles Jefferson & Abel Moore

# More Books by Charles Jefferson

Scan this QR code to discover more of Charles Jefferson's books on Amazon

.

# Table of Contents

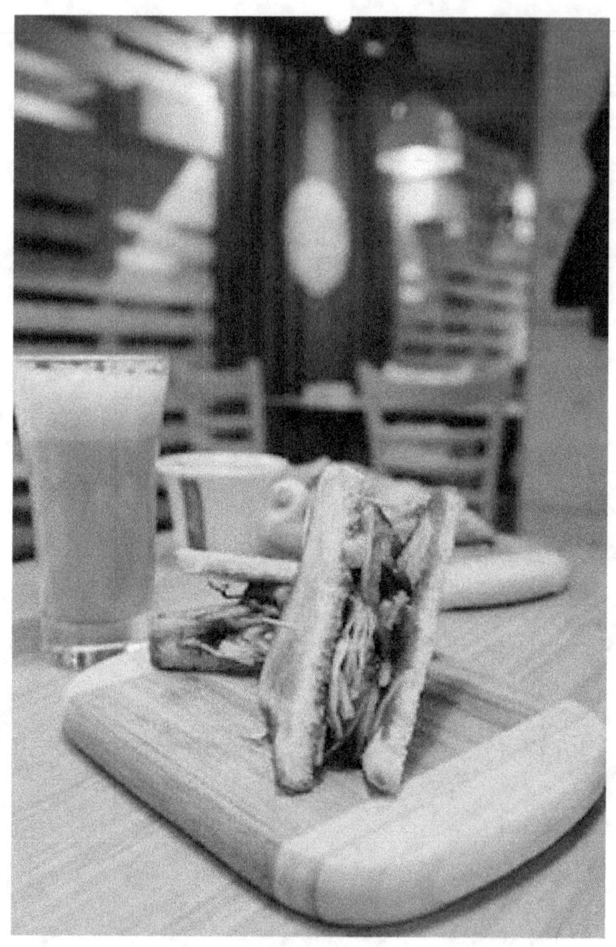

# Introduction



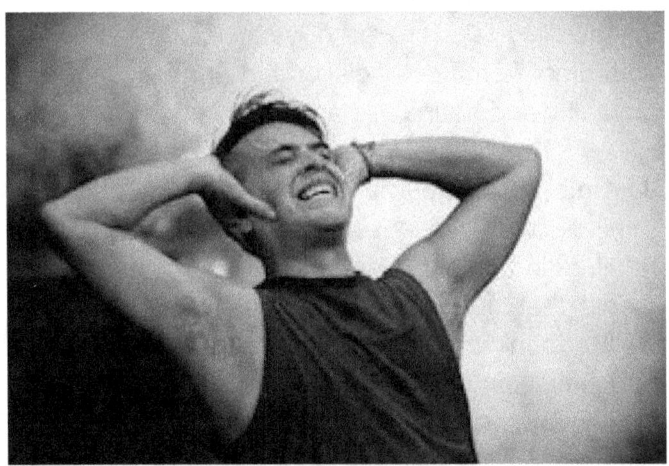

Welcome to "The Anti-Inflammatory Diet Cookbook for Beginners," your essential guide to unlocking the transformative power of food for optimal health and vitality. Within these pages, you'll discover how simple dietary changes can combat inflammation, boost energy levels, and revitalize your overall well-being.

Inflammation is more than just a nuisance; it's a silent driver of chronic disease lurking beneath the surface. But fear not, for you hold in your hands the key to reclaiming control over your health destiny. Through the strategic selection of anti-inflammatory foods and lifestyle practices, you have the power to silence inflammation and unleash your body's innate healing potential.

This book isn't just about recipes; it's a roadmap to a life brimming with vitality and abundance. It's an invitation to take charge of your health and rewrite your story from one of discomfort and fatigue to one of vitality and boundless energy.

Join me on this journey as we explore the science behind inflammation, stock our kitchens with healing ingredients, and whip up mouthwatering meals that nourish the body and soul. Together, we'll debunk myths, uncover hidden health truths, and empower you to make informed choices that propel you towards your health goals.

Are you ready to embrace a life free from inflammation's grip? Are you ready to step into your power and reclaim your vitality? If so, then let's embark on this transformative journey together. Your body deserves nothing less than the very best, and it all starts with what you put on your plate.

So, grab your apron, sharpen your knives, and prepare to embark on a culinary adventure that will change your life forever. Your journey to vibrant health starts now.

Charles Jefferson

# CHAPTER ONE

## Understanding Inflammation

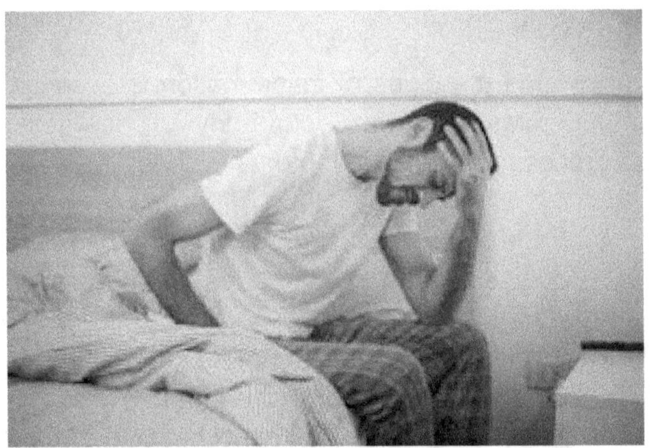

Inflammation is a natural process that occurs in the body as a response to injury or infection. While it's a vital part of the immune system's defense mechanism, chronic inflammation can have detrimental effects on health, leading to various diseases and conditions. In this chapter, we'll delve into the basics of inflammation, helping you understand what it is, why your body gets inflamed, and what happens during an inflammation.

## What is Inflammation?

At its core, inflammation is the body's way of protecting itself from harmful stimuli, such as pathogens, toxins, or physical injury. When tissue is damaged or infected, the immune system springs into action, triggering a cascade of biochemical processes to repair the damage and fend off invaders.

## Signs of Inflammation

Recognizing the signs of inflammation is essential for understanding when your body is undergoing this process. Common symptoms include:

- Redness: Increased blood flow to the affected area can cause redness and warmth.
- Swelling: Accumulation of fluid and immune cells leads to swelling or edema.
- Pain: Sensory nerves become more sensitive during inflammation, resulting in pain or discomfort.
- Heat: The increased metabolic activity in inflamed tissues can raise the temperature.

# The Role of Diet in Inflammation Management

Diet plays a crucial role in modulating inflammation levels in the body. Certain foods can either promote or reduce inflammation, making dietary choices a powerful tool in managing chronic inflammation.

## Foods That Promote Inflammation

A diet high in processed foods, refined sugars, unhealthy fats, and artificial additives can fuel inflammation in the body. These pro-inflammatory foods include:

- Refined carbohydrates: White bread, pastries, and sugary snacks can spike blood sugar levels and trigger inflammation.
- Trans fats: Found in fried foods, baked goods, and margarine, trans fats promote inflammation and increase the risk of chronic diseases.
- Sugary beverages: Soft drinks, fruit juices, and energy drinks are loaded with sugar, contributing to inflammation and insulin resistance.
- Processed meats: Deli meats, hot dogs, and bacon contain high levels of saturated fats and preservatives linked to inflammation and heart disease.

## Foods That Fight Inflammation

Conversely, adopting an anti-inflammatory diet rich in whole, nutrient-dense foods can help reduce inflammation and support overall health. These anti-inflammatory foods include:

- Fatty fish: Salmon, mackerel, and sardines are rich in omega-3 fatty acids, which have potent anti-inflammatory effects.

- Fruits and vegetables: Colourful fruits and veggies are packed with antioxidants and phytochemicals that combat inflammation and oxidative stress.
- Nuts and seeds: Almonds, walnuts, flaxseeds, and chia seeds are excellent sources of healthy fats, fiber, and anti-inflammatory compounds.
- Whole grains: Quinoa, brown rice, and oats provide fiber and nutrients that promote gut health and reduce inflammation.
- Herbs and spices: Turmeric, ginger, garlic, and cinnamon contain bioactive compounds with anti-inflammatory properties.

By making mindful food choices and prioritizing whole, unprocessed foods, you can help mitigate chronic inflammation and promote overall well-being. In the next section, we'll delve deeper into the mechanisms behind inflammation and explore how it impacts the body.

## Understanding the Mechanisms of Inflammation

To grasp the intricacies of inflammation, it's essential to understand the underlying biological processes that occur within the body.

## The Inflammatory Response

When tissue damage or infection occurs, the immune system releases signaling molecules called cytokines. These cytokines act as messengers, rallying immune cells to the site of injury or infection. White blood cells, such as neutrophils and macrophages, then engulf and destroy pathogens or damaged cells, initiating the inflammatory response.

## Acute vs. Chronic Inflammation

Inflammation can be categorised into two main types: acute and chronic. Acute inflammation is a short-term, localised response to injury or infection. It typically resolves once the underlying cause is eliminated or neutralised.

On the other hand, chronic inflammation is a persistent, low-grade inflammatory state that can linger for weeks, months, or even years. Unlike acute inflammation, which serves a protective role, chronic inflammation can contribute to the development of various chronic diseases, including heart disease, diabetes, cancer, and autoimmune disorders.

## Factors Contributing to Chronic Inflammation

Several factors can contribute to the development of chronic inflammation:

- Poor diet: A diet high in processed foods, refined sugars, and unhealthy fats can promote chronic inflammation.
- Lack of exercise: Sedentary behaviour and a lack of physical activity can exacerbate inflammation and impair immune function.
- Obesity: Excess body fat, especially visceral fat around the abdomen, produces inflammatory substances that contribute to chronic inflammation.
- Stress: Chronic stress can dysregulate the immune system and promote inflammation through the release of stress hormones like cortisol.
- Smoking: Tobacco smoke contains numerous toxins and chemicals that trigger inflammation and damage tissues throughout the body.

## Conclusion

Inflammation is a complex biological process that plays a crucial role in the body's defense against infection and injury. However, when inflammation becomes chronic, it can have detrimental effects on health and contribute to the development of various diseases.

By adopting an anti-inflammatory diet rich in whole, nutrient-dense foods and implementing lifestyle changes that promote overall well-being, you can help mitigate chronic inflammation and support optimal health. Understanding the basics of inflammation and its impact on the body is the first step toward living a healthier, more vibrant life.

In the next sections of our "Anti-Inflammatory Diet Cookbook for Beginners," we'll explore practical strategies for to prepare you for a war against anti inflammation

Remember, small changes can yield significant results when it comes to inflammation management. Stay tuned for more expert advice and actionable tips on your journey to wellness.

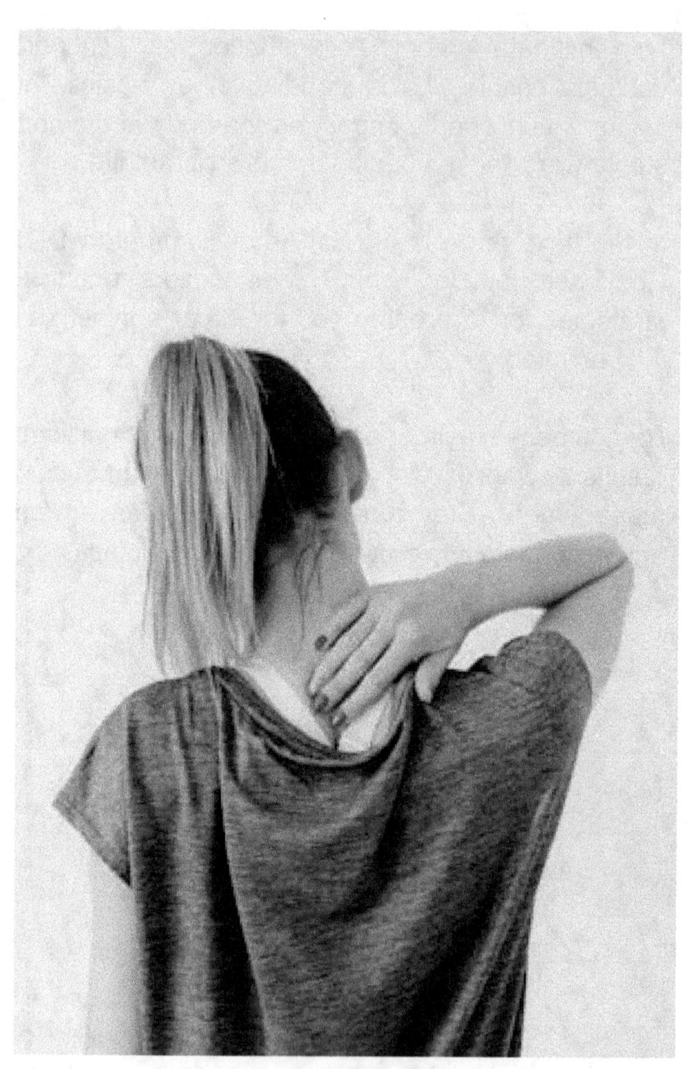

# CHAPTER TWO

## Getting Started with the Anti-Inflammatory Diet

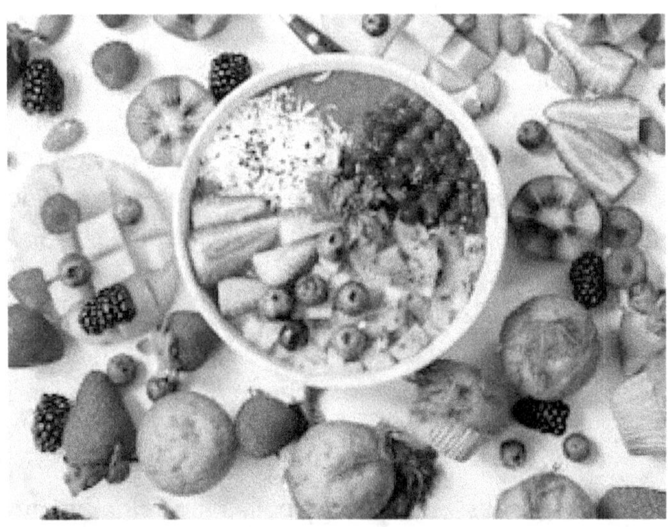

In today's fast-paced world, many individuals find themselves grappling with various health challenges, among which inflammation ranks high. Whether it's joint pain, digestive issues, or persistent fatigue, inflammation can significantly impact one's quality of life. However, there's hope on the horizon in the form of an anti-inflammatory diet.

# Preparing Your Kitchen

Equipping your kitchen with the necessary tools and ingredients is fundamental to embracing an anti-inflammatory diet. Here's how you can set yourself up for success:

## Essential Tools:

- Quality Blender: Invest in a high-powered blender capable of pulverising fruits, vegetables, and nuts into smooth, creamy textures. A blender is essential for creating nutrient-packed smoothies, sauces, and soups that form the backbone of an anti-inflammatory diet.
- Food Processor: A food processor is a versatile tool for chopping, slicing, and shredding ingredients with precision. It's perfect for preparing homemade dips, spreads, and energy balls using wholesome ingredients like nuts, seeds, and dried fruits.
- Juicer: While not essential, a juicer can be a valuable addition to your kitchen arsenal, especially if you enjoy fresh fruit and vegetable juices. Juicing allows you to extract concentrated doses of vitamins, minerals, and antioxidants from produce, providing a convenient way to boost your intake of anti-inflammatory nutrients.
- Immersion Blender: Also known as a hand blender, an immersion blender is a handy tool for blending soups, sauces, and

smoothies directly in the pot or container. Its compact size and easy cleanup make it a practical choice for smaller kitchens or quick meal preparation.

- Steamer Basket: Steaming is a gentle cooking method that helps preserve the nutrients and flavours of vegetables without added fats or oils. Invest in a quality steamer basket or steaming insert for your pots to effortlessly cook a variety of vegetables for your anti-inflammatory meals.
- Vegetable Spiralizer: For a fun and creative way to incorporate more vegetables into your diet, consider investing in a vegetable spiralizer. This tool allows you to transform zucchini, carrots, and other vegetables into noodle-like strands, perfect for replacing traditional pasta in anti-inflammatory recipes.
- Mortar and Pestle: Grinding herbs and spices fresh just before use releases their essential oils and maximises their flavour and nutritional benefits. A mortar and pestle are essential tools for crushing herbs, grinding spices, and creating flavorful spice blends to elevate your anti-inflammatory dishes.
- Measuring Cups and Spoons: Accurate measurement of ingredients is crucial for achieving consistent results in cooking and baking. Invest in a set of durable measuring

cups and spoons to ensure precise portioning of anti-inflammatory ingredients in your recipes.

- Herb Stripper: This handy tool makes quick work of stripping herbs like rosemary, thyme, and parsley from their stems, saving you time and effort in meal preparation. It ensures that you can easily incorporate fresh herbs into your anti-inflammatory dishes for added flavour and nutritional benefits.

- Citrus Juicer: Freshly squeezed citrus juice adds brightness and acidity to dishes, enhancing their flavour profile. A citrus juicer allows you to extract every last drop of juice from lemons, limes, oranges, and grapefruits, making it easier to incorporate these immune-boosting fruits into your anti-inflammatory diet.

- Salad Spinner: Washing and drying leafy greens and herbs is essential for crisp and vibrant salads. A salad spinner removes excess water from washed greens, ensuring that your salads are not waterlogged and maintaining their freshness for longer periods.

- Microplane Grater/Zester: A microplane grater or zester is a versatile tool for grating citrus zest, garlic, ginger, and hard cheeses like Parmesan. It allows you to add intense flavour to your dishes with minimal effort and is essential for incorporating aromatic ingredients into your anti-inflammatory recipes.

- Kitchen Timer: Precision timing is crucial for achieving perfect results in cooking and baking. A reliable kitchen timer helps you keep track of cooking times and ensures that your anti-inflammatory dishes are cooked to perfection without overcooking or undercooking.
- Cutting Boards: Invest in high-quality cutting boards made from durable materials like bamboo or plastic. Having multiple cutting boards in different sizes ensures that you can designate specific boards for cutting raw meat, poultry, fish, and vegetables, reducing the risk of cross-contamination.
- Strainer or Colander: Straining liquids, rinsing grains, and draining cooked pasta or vegetables are common tasks in meal preparation. A strainer or colander with fine mesh allows you to efficiently separate solids from liquids and ensures that your anti-inflammatory dishes are free from excess moisture.
- Kitchen Shears: Kitchen shears are versatile tools for trimming herbs, cutting parchment paper, and even spatchcocking poultry. They offer precision and control in meal preparation, making them indispensable for any home cook embracing an anti-inflammatory diet.

By equipping your kitchen with these essential tools, you'll be well-equipped to embark on your anti-inflammatory diet journey with confidence and culinary creativity. Experiment with different recipes, flavours, and cooking techniques to discover the delicious and nourishing possibilities of anti-inflammatory eating.

## Essential Ingredients:

- Colourful Fruits and Vegetables: Fill your fridge and pantry with an array of vibrant fruits and vegetables, such as berries, leafy greens, tomatoes, carrots, and sweet potatoes. These plant-based foods are rich in antioxidants and phytonutrients, which combat inflammation and support overall health.
- Healthy Fats: Incorporate sources of healthy fats into your diet, including avocados, extra virgin olive oil, nuts, and seeds. These fats contain omega-3 fatty acids and monounsaturated fats, which possess anti-inflammatory properties and promote heart health.
- Lean Proteins: Choose lean protein sources such as poultry, fish, tofu, tempeh, and legumes to fuel your body with essential amino acids. These proteins aid in muscle repair and support immune function without contributing to inflammation.

- Whole Grains: Opt for whole grains like quinoa, brown rice, oats, and barley over refined grains. Whole grains are rich in fiber, vitamins, and minerals, promoting digestive health and providing sustained energy levels.
- Herbs and Spices: Enhance the flavor of your meals with herbs and spices known for their anti-inflammatory properties. Turmeric, ginger, garlic, cinnamon, and cayenne pepper are excellent additions that not only add depth to dishes but also offer health benefits.
- Dark Chocolate: Indulge in dark chocolate with a high cocoa content (70% or higher) as an occasional treat. Dark chocolate contains flavonoids and antioxidants that have anti-inflammatory effects and may benefit heart health.
- Probiotic Foods: Incorporate probiotic-rich foods like yoghourt, kefir, sauerkraut, kimchi, and kombucha into your diet. These fermented foods contain beneficial bacteria that support gut health and reduce inflammation in the body.
- Legumes: Include a variety of legumes such as lentils, chickpeas, black beans, and kidney beans in your anti-inflammatory meals. Legumes are rich in fiber, protein, and antioxidants that help lower inflammation and promote digestive health.

- Berries: Stock up on antioxidant-rich berries like blueberries, strawberries, raspberries, and blackberries. These delicious fruits are packed with vitamins, minerals, and phytochemicals that help combat inflammation and protect against chronic diseases.

## Setting Realistic Goals:

Embarking on an anti-inflammatory diet journey requires patience, commitment, and realistic goal-setting. Here are some tips to help you stay on track:

- Start Gradually: Introduce changes to your diet gradually rather than attempting a complete overhaul overnight. Focus on incorporating one new anti-inflammatory food or recipe each week.
- Educate Yourself: Take the time to learn about the principles of anti-inflammatory eating and the benefits of specific foods. Understanding the science behind your dietary choices can reinforce your commitment and motivation.
- Listen to Your Body: Pay attention to how different foods make you feel. Keep a food diary to track your symptoms and identify potential triggers of inflammation.
- Seek Support: Surround yourself with supportive friends, family members, or

online communities who share your health goals. Having a support system can provide encouragement, accountability, and practical tips for navigating challenges.

By equipping your kitchen with essential tools and ingredients and setting realistic goals, you're laying the foundation for success on your anti-inflammatory journey. In the next section, we'll address common challenges faced by individuals managing inflammation and provide strategies to overcome them.

## Overcoming Common Challenges

While adopting an anti-inflammatory diet can yield numerous health benefits, it's not without its challenges. Here are some common hurdles individuals may encounter along the way and strategies to overcome them:

- Social Situations
    - Challenge: Dining out or attending social gatherings where unhealthy food choices are prevalent can make sticking to an anti-inflammatory diet difficult.
    - Strategy: Plan ahead by reviewing restaurant menus online and choosing establishments with healthier options. Offer to bring a dish to potlucks or gatherings that aligns with your dietary preferences.

- Cravings and Temptations:
    - Challenge: Cravings for sugary snacks, processed foods, or comfort foods can derail your anti-inflammatory efforts.
    - Strategy: Stock your kitchen with satisfying alternatives like fresh fruit, nuts, or dark chocolate. Practise mindful eating to recognize true hunger cues and differentiate between cravings and genuine hunger.
- Time Constraints:
    - Challenge: Busy schedules and time constraints may lead to relying on convenience foods or skipping meals altogether.
    - Strategy: Prioritise meal planning and batch cooking on weekends to have nutritious meals readily available during the week. Utilize slow cookers, pressure cookers, or meal delivery services to streamline the cooking process.
- Budgetary Constraints:
    - Challenge: The perception that healthy eating is expensive may deter individuals from purchasing nutrient-dense foods.
    - Strategy: Shop smart by buying seasonal produce, opting for frozen

or canned fruits and vegetables when fresh options are cost-prohibitive, and buying in bulk to save money. Focus on purchasing whole foods rather than processed or packaged items.

- Family Preferences:
  - Challenge: Family members may have different dietary preferences or be resistant to trying new foods.
  - Strategy: Involve family members in meal planning and preparation to increase buy-in and accommodate individual preferences. Introduce new foods gradually and offer a variety of options to cater to different tastes.

- Emotional Eating:
  - Challenge: Using food as a coping mechanism for stress, boredom, or emotional distress can lead to overeating or making unhealthy food choices.
  - Strategy: Practice stress-reduction techniques such as deep breathing, meditation, or engaging in hobbies to manage emotions without turning to food. Seek support from a therapist or counsellor if emotional eating becomes a recurring issue.

By anticipating and addressing these common challenges, you can navigate your anti-inflammatory diet journey with confidence and resilience. Remember that progress is a journey, not a destination, and every positive choice you make contributes to your overall well-being. In the following sections, we'll explore specific meal ideas and recipes to help you incorporate anti-inflammatory foods into your daily routine.

# CHAPTER THREE

## Anti-Inflammatory Diet Meal Planning

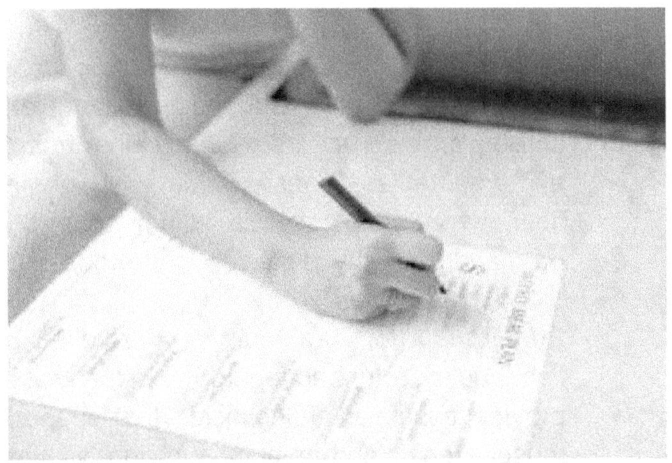

Inflammation is the body's natural response to injury or infection, but when it becomes chronic, it can lead to various health issues such as heart disease, arthritis, and even cancer. Fortunately, one powerful way to combat chronic inflammation is through diet. By incorporating anti-inflammatory foods into your meals and avoiding pro-inflammatory ones, you can help reduce inflammation in your body and improve your overall health.

# Macronutrients and Micronutrients

When planning an anti-inflammatory diet, it's essential to focus on both macronutrients (carbohydrates, protein, and fat) and micronutrients (vitamins and minerals). Here's a breakdown of each:

## Macronutrients

- Carbohydrates: Choose complex carbohydrates such as whole grains, fruits, and vegetables. These foods are high in fiber, which helps reduce inflammation by promoting healthy digestion and stabilizing blood sugar levels.
- Protein: Opt for lean sources of protein like fish, poultry, tofu, and legumes. These foods provide essential amino acids that support muscle repair and immune function without adding excess saturated fat, which can contribute to inflammation.
- Healthy Fats: Incorporate sources of omega-3 fatty acids such as salmon, walnuts, and flaxseeds. Omega-3s have powerful anti-inflammatory properties and can help balance the omega-6 fatty acids found in many processed foods, which tend to promote inflammation.

## Micronutrients

- Vitamins: Ensure you're getting plenty of vitamins A, C, D, and E, as well as B vitamins like folate and B12. These vitamins play crucial roles in immune function and have anti-inflammatory effects.
- Minerals: Focus on minerals such as magnesium, zinc, and selenium, which have antioxidant properties and help reduce inflammation. Green leafy vegetables, nuts, seeds, and seafood are excellent sources of these minerals.

# Sample Meal Plans

Here's a sample meal plan for a day that incorporates anti-inflammatory foods:

## Breakfast:

- Spinach and Mushroom Omelette*: Spinach is rich in vitamins A and C, while mushrooms provide selenium. Eggs offer high-quality protein and healthy fats.
- Whole Grain Toast: Choose whole grain bread for added fiber and nutrients.

## Lunch:

- Grilled Salmon Salad: Salmon is a great source of omega-3 fatty acids. Pair it with leafy greens, tomatoes, cucumbers, and avocado for a nutritious and satisfying meal.

- Quinoa:
  Quinoa is a complete protein and contains anti-inflammatory compounds like quercetin.

**Dinner:**

- Mixed Berries: Berries are packed with antioxidants and can help reduce inflammation.

## Tips for Grocery Shopping and Meal Prepping

Now that you have an idea of what foods to include in your anti-inflammatory diet, let's discuss some tips to make grocery shopping and meal prepping easier and more cost-effective:

- Plan Ahead: Before heading to the grocery store, take some time to plan your meals for the week. This will help you create a shopping list and avoid impulse purchases of unhealthy foods.
- Focus on Fresh Produce: Stock up on a variety of fruits and vegetables, aiming for a colorful selection. Fresh produce is rich in vitamins, minerals, and antioxidants, all of which can help reduce inflammation.
- Choose Whole Grains: When selecting grains, opt for whole grains like brown rice, quinoa, and oats. These grains are higher in fiber and nutrients compared to refined

grains, which have been stripped of their nutritional content.

- Shop the Perimeter: In most grocery stores, the perimeter is where you'll find fresh produce, meats, and dairy products. Try to spend the majority of your time shopping in these areas and limit your exposure to processed foods found in the inner aisles.
- Read Labels: When purchasing packaged foods, read the ingredient list and nutrition label carefully. Look for products with minimal added sugars, unhealthy fats, and artificial ingredients. Choose items with recognizable, whole food ingredients.
- Buy in Bulk: Consider buying staple items like grains, beans, nuts, and seeds in bulk to save money and reduce packaging waste. Just be sure to store them properly in airtight containers to maintain freshness.
- Meal Prep in Batches: Set aside time each week to prepare large batches of staple foods like grains, proteins, and vegetables. This will make it easier to throw together healthy meals throughout the week, saving you time and reducing the temptation to order takeout.
- Experiment with Herbs and Spices: Enhance the flavor of your meals without adding extra salt or unhealthy sauces by experimenting with herbs and spices. Many herbs and spices, such as turmeric, ginger, and garlic, have anti-inflammatory

properties and can elevate the nutritional value of your dishes.

By following these tips, you can streamline your shopping and meal prep process while supporting your anti-inflammatory diet goals. Remember to listen to your body and make adjustments as needed to find what works best for you. Stay tuned for more expert advice on how to optimize your diet for inflammation relief.

## Conclusion

Incorporating an anti-inflammatory diet into your lifestyle can have profound effects on your health and well-being. By focusing on nutrient-dense foods rich in vitamins, minerals, antioxidants, and omega-3 fatty acids, you can help reduce inflammation in your body and lower your risk of chronic diseases.

Remember that meal planning is just one part of the equation. Pairing your nutritious meals with regular physical activity, stress management techniques, and adequate sleep can further enhance the anti-inflammatory benefits of your diet.

As you embark on your anti-inflammatory journey, be patient with yourself and celebrate small victories along the way. Every positive food choice you make is a step toward better health and vitality.

Stay informed, stay committed, and stay well. Here's to a life of vibrant health and vitality through the power of anti-inflammatory nutrition.

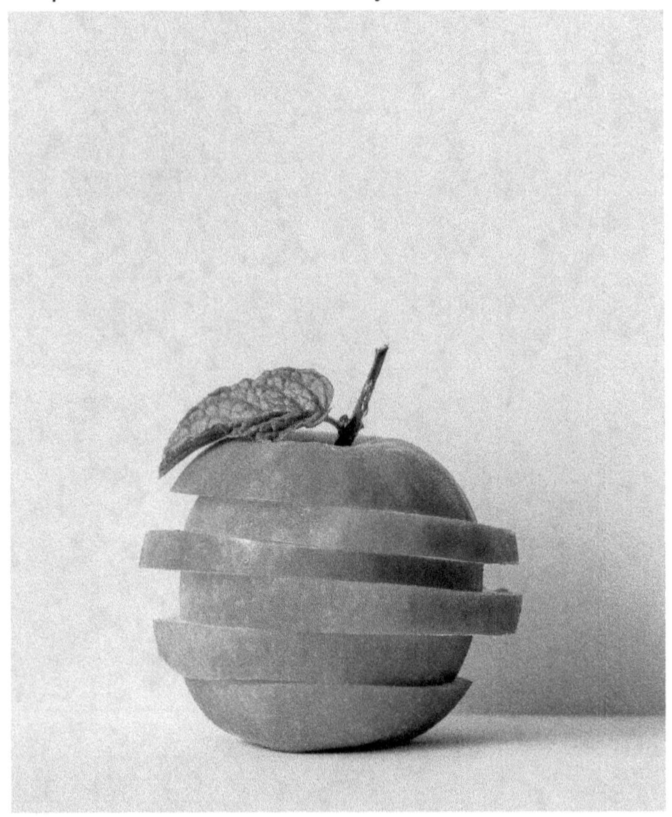

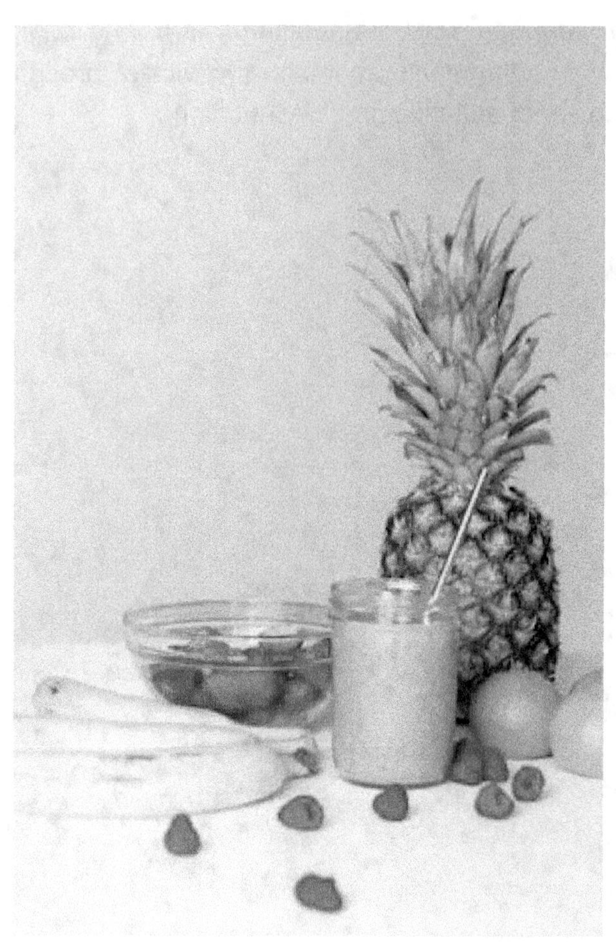

# CHAPTER FOUR

## Soups

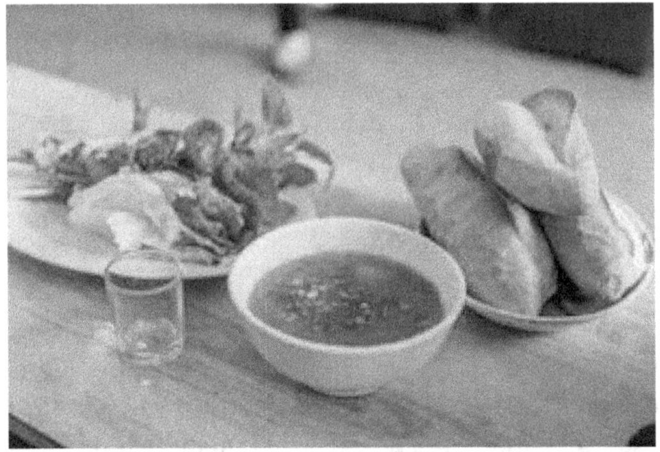

Soups have long been hailed as a comfort food, offering warmth, nourishment, and a sense of well-being. But did you know that soups can also play a crucial role in managing inflammation and promoting overall health? In this chapter, we will explore 15 delicious and nutritious soup recipes specifically designed to combat inflammation and support healing.

# Why Soups?

Soups provide an excellent opportunity to pack a wide array of anti-inflammatory ingredients into one delicious bowl. From vibrant vegetables to healing herbs and spices, each ingredient contributes to reducing inflammation and supporting the body's natural healing processes.

One of the best things about soups is their versatility. Whether you prefer creamy pureed soups, chunky vegetable-packed stews, or spicy chili, there's a soup recipe to suit every palate and dietary preference. Don't be afraid to get creative with your ingredients and experiment with different flavor combinations to find what works best for you.

By simmering ingredients together, soups allow for the flavors to meld and develop, creating a comforting and nourishing meal that is both satisfying and healing. Whether you're experiencing chronic inflammation or simply looking to support your overall health, incorporating anti-inflammatory soups into your diet can be a powerful strategy.

In the following sections, we'll dive into 15 delicious anti-inflammatory soup recipes, complete with ingredient lists, US measurements, and step-by-step instructions for preparation. Each recipe is carefully crafted to nourish your body, soothe inflammation, and delight your taste buds. So, let's get cooking and experience the healing power of soups firsthand

# Turmeric Carrot Soup

## Ingredients:

- 1 tablespoon olive oil
- 1 onion, diced
- 3 cloves garlic, minced
- 1 tablespoon grated fresh ginger
- 1 teaspoon ground turmeric
- 4 cups chopped carrots
- 4 cups vegetable broth
- Salt and pepper, to taste
- Coconut milk (optional, for garnish)
- Fresh cilantro (optional, for garnish)

## Procedure:

1. Heat olive oil in a large pot over medium heat. Add diced onion and cook until softened, about 5 minutes.
2. Add minced garlic, grated ginger, and ground turmeric to the pot. Cook for an additional 2 minutes, stirring frequently.
3. Add chopped carrots and vegetable broth to the pot. Bring to a boil, then reduce heat and simmer until carrots are tender, about 20 minutes.
4. Use an immersion blender to puree the soup until smooth. Alternatively, transfer the soup to a blender and puree in batches.

5. Season with salt and pepper to taste. If desired, swirl in a splash of coconut milk for added creaminess and garnish with fresh cilantro before serving.

This vibrant Turmeric Carrot Soup is not only bursting with flavor but also packed with anti-inflammatory ingredients like turmeric and ginger. Enjoy a comforting bowl of this soup to soothe inflammation and nourish your body from the inside out.

## Spinach and White Bean Soup

**Ingredients**:
- 1 tablespoon olive oil
- 1 onion, diced
- 3 cloves garlic, minced
- 1 teaspoon dried thyme
- 4 cups vegetable broth
- 2 cans (15 ounces each) white beans, drained and rinsed
- 4 cups chopped spinach
- Salt and pepper, to taste
- Lemon wedges (optional, for serving)

**Procedure:**
1. Heat olive oil in a large pot over medium heat. Add diced onion and cook until translucent, about 5 minutes.

2. Add minced garlic and dried thyme to the pot. Cook for an additional 2 minutes, stirring frequently.
3. Pour vegetable broth into the pot and bring to a simmer.
4. Add white beans and chopped spinach to the pot. Simmer for 10-15 minutes, until the spinach is wilted and the flavors are well combined.
5. Season with salt and pepper to taste. Serve hot with a squeeze of fresh lemon juice, if desired.

This Spinach and White Bean Soup is a nourishing and comforting dish that's perfect for supporting inflammation management. Packed with fiber-rich beans and nutrient-dense spinach, it's a wholesome meal that will leave you feeling satisfied and nourished.

## Butternut Squash and Ginger Soup

**Ingredients:**
- 1 tablespoon coconut oil
- 1 onion, diced
- 3 cloves garlic, minced
- 1 tablespoon grated fresh ginger
- 1 medium butternut squash, peeled, seeded, and diced
- 4 cups vegetable broth
- 1 (13.5-ounce) can coconut milk
- Salt and pepper, to taste

- Fresh cilantro (optional, for garnish)

## Procedure:

1. In a large pot, heat coconut oil over medium heat. Add diced onion and cook until softened, about 5 minutes.
2. Add minced garlic and grated ginger to the pot. Cook for another 2 minutes, stirring frequently.
3. Add diced butternut squash and vegetable broth to the pot. Bring to a boil, then reduce heat and simmer until squash is tender, about 20 minutes.
4. Use an immersion blender to puree the soup until smooth. Alternatively, transfer the soup to a blender and puree in batches.
5. Stir in coconut milk and season with salt and pepper to taste. Simmer for an additional 5 minutes to heat through.
6. Serve hot, garnished with fresh cilantro if desired.

Butternut Squash and Ginger Soup is a velvety-smooth and comforting dish that's perfect for chilly days. Packed with beta-carotene-rich butternut squash and anti-inflammatory ginger, this soup is a flavorful way to support your body's natural healing processes.

# Lentil and Kale Soup

**Ingredients:**
- 1 tablespoon olive oil
- 1 onion, diced
- 2 carrots, diced
- 2 stalks celery, diced
- 3 cloves garlic, minced
- 1 teaspoon ground cumin
- 1 teaspoon smoked paprika
- 1 cup dried green lentils, rinsed and drained
- 6 cups vegetable broth
- 4 cups chopped kale
- Salt and pepper, to taste
- Lemon wedges (optional, for serving)

**Procedure:**
1. Heat olive oil in a large pot over medium heat. Add diced onion, carrots, and celery. Cook until vegetables are softened, about 5-7 minutes.
2. Add minced garlic, ground cumin, and smoked paprika to the pot. Cook for an additional 2 minutes, stirring frequently.
3. Add dried green lentils and vegetable broth to the pot. Bring to a boil, then reduce heat and simmer until lentils are tender, about 20-25 minutes.

4. Stir in chopped kale and simmer for an additional 5 minutes, until kale is wilted.
5. Season with salt and pepper to taste. Serve hot with a squeeze of fresh lemon juice, if desired.

Lentil and Kale Soup is a hearty and nutritious dish that's perfect for satisfying your hunger and supporting inflammation management. Packed with protein-rich lentils and nutrient-dense kale, this soup is a delicious way to nourish your body and promote overall health.

## Tomato Basil Soup

**Ingredients:**
- 1 tablespoon olive oil
- 1 onion, diced
- 3 cloves garlic, minced
- 2 cans (28 ounces each) diced tomatoes
- 1 tablespoon tomato paste
- 4 cups vegetable broth
- 1 teaspoon dried basil
- Salt and pepper, to taste
- Fresh basil leaves (optional, for garnish)

**Procedure:**
1. Heat olive oil in a large pot over medium heat. Add diced onion and cook until softened, about 5 minutes.
2. Add minced garlic to the pot and cook for another 2 minutes, stirring frequently.

3. Add diced tomatoes, tomato paste, vegetable broth, and dried basil to the pot. Bring to a boil, then reduce heat and simmer for 20-25 minutes.
4. Use an immersion blender to puree the soup until smooth. Alternatively, transfer the soup to a blender and puree in batches.
5. Season with salt and pepper to taste. Serve hot, garnished with fresh basil leaves if desired.

Tomato Basil Soup is a classic comfort food with a twist of anti-inflammatory goodness. Tomatoes are rich in lycopene, a powerful antioxidant that helps combat inflammation, while basil adds flavor and freshness. Enjoy a bowl of this soup for a comforting and nourishing meal.

## Quinoa Vegetable Soup

**Ingredients:**
- 1 tablespoon olive oil
- 1 onion, diced
- 2 carrots, diced
- 2 stalks celery, diced
- 3 cloves garlic, minced
- 1 cup quinoa, rinsed
- 6 cups vegetable broth
- 2 cups chopped mixed vegetables (such as bell peppers, zucchini, and mushrooms)
- Salt and pepper, to taste
- Fresh parsley (optional, for garnish)

**Procedure:**

1. Heat olive oil in a large pot over medium heat. Add diced onion, carrots, and celery. Cook until vegetables are softened, about 5-7 minutes.
2. Add minced garlic to the pot and cook for another 2 minutes, stirring frequently.
3. Add quinoa and vegetable broth to the pot. Bring to a boil, then reduce heat and simmer for 15 minutes.
4. Stir in chopped mixed vegetables and simmer for an additional 10-15 minutes, until quinoa and vegetables are tender.
5. Season with salt and pepper to taste. Serve hot, garnished with fresh parsley if desired.

Quinoa Vegetable Soup is a hearty and satisfying dish that's perfect for nourishing your body and supporting inflammation management. Quinoa is a complete protein and a good source of fiber, while the mixed vegetables add flavor and nutritional value. Enjoy a bowl of this soup for a wholesome and comforting meal.

## Ginger Garlic Miso Soup

**Ingredients:**

- 4 cups vegetable broth
- 2 tablespoons white miso paste
- 2 cloves garlic, minced
- 1 tablespoon grated fresh ginger

- 1 cup sliced shiitake mushrooms
- 2 green onions, thinly sliced
- 1 cup chopped spinach
- 1 tablespoon soy sauce
- 1 teaspoon sesame oil
- Red pepper flakes (optional, for garnish)

## Procedure:

1. In a large pot, bring vegetable broth to a simmer over medium heat.
2. In a small bowl, whisk together miso paste and a ladleful of hot broth until smooth.
3. Add minced garlic, grated ginger, sliced shiitake mushrooms, and chopped spinach to the pot. Simmer for 5-7 minutes until mushrooms are tender.
4. Stir in sliced green onions, soy sauce, and sesame oil. Simmer for an additional 2-3 minutes.
5. Taste and adjust seasoning as needed. Serve hot, garnished with red pepper flakes if desired.

Ginger Garlic Miso Soup is a comforting and flavorful dish that's perfect for supporting inflammation management. Miso paste adds depth of flavor and beneficial probiotics, while ginger and garlic provide anti-inflammatory properties. Enjoy a bowl of this soup for a nourishing and satisfying meal.

# Coconut Curry Lentil Soup

## Ingredients:

- 1 tablespoon coconut oil
- 1 onion, diced
- 3 cloves garlic, minced
- 1 tablespoon grated fresh ginger
- 1 tablespoon curry powder
- 1 cup dried red lentils, rinsed
- 4 cups vegetable broth
- 1 (13.5-ounce) can coconut milk
- 2 cups chopped kale
- Salt and pepper, to taste
- Fresh cilantro (optional, for garnish)

## Procedure:

1. In a large pot, heat coconut oil over medium heat. Add diced onion and cook until softened, about 5 minutes.
2. Add minced garlic, grated ginger, and curry powder to the pot. Cook for an additional 2 minutes, stirring frequently.
3. Add dried red lentils and vegetable broth to the pot. Bring to a boil, then reduce heat and simmer for 15-20 minutes, until lentils are tender.
4. Stir in coconut milk and chopped kale. Simmer for an additional 5 minutes, until kale is wilted.
5. Season with salt and pepper to taste. Serve hot, garnished with fresh cilantro if desired.

Coconut Curry Lentil Soup is a flavorful and nourishing dish that's perfect for supporting inflammation management. Red lentils provide protein and fiber, while coconut milk adds creaminess and healthy fats. Enjoy a bowl of this soup for a satisfying and comforting meal.

# Roasted Red Pepper and Tomato Soup

## Ingredients:
- 3 large red bell peppers
- 2 tablespoons olive oil
- 1 onion, diced
- 3 cloves garlic, minced
- 1 (28-ounce) can diced tomatoes
- 4 cups vegetable broth
- 1 teaspoon dried thyme
- Salt and pepper, to taste
- Fresh basil leaves (optional, for garnish)

## Procedure:
1. Preheat the oven to 400°F (200°C). Line a baking sheet with parchment paper.
2. Place whole red bell peppers on the prepared baking sheet and roast in the preheated oven for 25-30 minutes, until the skins are charred and blistered.
3. Remove the roasted bell peppers from the oven and transfer them to a heatproof bowl.

Cover the bowl with plastic wrap and let the peppers steam for 10 minutes.

4.  Once cooled, peel off the charred skins from the roasted bell peppers and discard the seeds and stems. Chop the flesh into small pieces.
5.  In a large pot, heat olive oil over medium heat. Add diced onion and cook until softened, about 5 minutes.
6.  Add minced garlic to the pot and cook for another 2 minutes, stirring frequently.
7.  Add diced tomatoes (with their juices), roasted red peppers, vegetable broth, and dried thyme to the pot. Bring to a boil, then reduce heat and simmer for 15-20 minutes.
8.  Use an immersion blender to puree the soup until smooth. Alternatively, transfer the soup to a blender and puree in batches.
9.  Season with salt and pepper to taste. Serve hot, garnished with fresh basil leaves if desired.

Roasted Red Pepper and Tomato Soup is a flavorful and vibrant dish that's perfect for supporting inflammation management. Red bell peppers are rich in vitamin C and antioxidants, while tomatoes provide lycopene, a powerful anti-inflammatory compound. Enjoy a bowl of this soup for a comforting and nourishing meal.

# Sweet Potato and Kale Soup

## Ingredients:

- 1 tablespoon olive oil
- 1 onion, diced
- 2 cloves garlic, minced
- 2 medium sweet potatoes, peeled and diced
- 4 cups vegetable broth
- 2 cups chopped kale
- 1 (13.5-ounce) can coconut milk
- Salt and pepper, to taste
- Fresh parsley (optional, for garnish)

## Procedure:

1. In a large pot, heat olive oil over medium heat. Add diced onion and cook until softened, about 5 minutes.
2. Add minced garlic to the pot and cook for another 2 minutes, stirring frequently.
3. Add diced sweet potatoes and vegetable broth to the pot. Bring to a boil, then reduce heat and simmer for 15-20 minutes, until sweet potatoes are tender.
4. Use an immersion blender to puree the soup until smooth. Alternatively, transfer the soup to a blender and puree in batches.
5. Stir in chopped kale and coconut milk. Simmer for an additional 5 minutes, until kale is wilted and flavors are well combined.
6. Season with salt and pepper to taste. Serve hot, garnished with fresh parsley if desired.

Sweet Potato and Kale Soup is a hearty and nutritious dish that's perfect for supporting inflammation management. Sweet potatoes are rich in beta-carotene and vitamins, while kale adds fiber and essential nutrients. Enjoy a bowl of this soup for a satisfying and nourishing meal.

## Mushroom Barley Soup

### Ingredients:

- 1 tablespoon olive oil
- 1 onion, diced
- 2 carrots, diced
- 2 stalks celery, diced
- 8 ounces mushrooms, sliced
- 3 cloves garlic, minced
- 1 cup pearl barley
- 6 cups vegetable broth
- 1 teaspoon dried thyme
- Salt and pepper, to taste
- Fresh parsley (optional, for garnish)

### Procedure:

1. In a large pot, heat olive oil over medium heat. Add diced onion, carrots, and celery. Cook until vegetables are softened, about 5-7 minutes.
2. Add sliced mushrooms to the pot and cook for another 5 minutes, until mushrooms are tender.
3. Add minced garlic to the pot and cook for an additional 2 minutes, stirring frequently.

4. Stir in pearl barley and vegetable broth. Bring to a boil, then reduce heat and simmer for 30-40 minutes, until barley is tender.
5. Season with dried thyme, salt, and pepper to taste. Serve hot, garnished with fresh parsley if desired.

Mushroom Barley Soup is a hearty and comforting dish that's perfect for supporting inflammation management. Barley is a good source of fiber and selenium, while mushrooms provide antioxidants and immune-boosting properties. Enjoy a bowl of this soup for a nourishing and satisfying meal.

## Cauliflower and Leek Soup

**Ingredients:**
- 1 tablespoon olive oil
- 2 leeks, white and light green parts only, sliced
- 1 head cauliflower, chopped
- 3 cloves garlic, minced
- 4 cups vegetable broth
- 1 teaspoon dried thyme
- Salt and pepper, to taste
- Lemon zest (optional, for garnish)

**Procedure:**
1. In a large pot, heat olive oil over medium heat. Add sliced leeks and cook until softened, about 5 minutes.

2. Add chopped cauliflower to the pot and cook for another 5 minutes, until slightly golden.
3. Add minced garlic to the pot and cook for an additional 2 minutes, stirring frequently.
4. Pour vegetable broth into the pot and bring to a boil. Reduce heat and simmer for 20-25 minutes, until cauliflower is tender.
5. Use an immersion blender to puree the soup until smooth. Alternatively, transfer the soup to a blender and puree in batches.
6. Season with dried thyme, salt, and pepper to taste. Serve hot, garnished with lemon zest if desired.

Cauliflower and Leek Soup is a creamy and flavorful dish that's perfect for supporting inflammation management. Cauliflower is rich in antioxidants and vitamin C, while leeks add a subtle sweetness and depth of flavor. Enjoy a bowl of this soup for a nourishing and comforting meal.

## Broccoli and Turmeric Soup

### Ingredients:
- 1 tablespoon olive oil
- 1 onion, diced
- 3 cloves garlic, minced
- 1 head broccoli, chopped
- 1 teaspoon ground turmeric
- 4 cups vegetable broth
- 1 cup coconut milk

- Salt and pepper, to taste
- Lemon wedges (optional, for serving)

## Procedure:

1. In a large pot, heat olive oil over medium heat. Add diced onion and cook until softened, about 5 minutes.
2. Add minced garlic to the pot and cook for another 2 minutes, stirring frequently.
3. Add chopped broccoli and ground turmeric to the pot. Cook for 5 minutes, stirring occasionally.
4. Pour vegetable broth into the pot and bring to a boil. Reduce heat and simmer for 15-20 minutes, until broccoli is tender.
5. Use an immersion blender to puree the soup until smooth. Alternatively, transfer the soup to a blender and puree in batches.
6. Stir in coconut milk and season with salt and pepper to taste. Simmer for an additional 5 minutes.
7. Serve hot, with lemon wedges on the side for squeezing over the soup if desired.

Broccoli and Turmeric Soup is a nutritious and flavorful dish that's perfect for supporting inflammation management. Broccoli is rich in antioxidants and fiber, while turmeric provides anti-inflammatory properties. Enjoy a bowl of this soup for a nourishing and comforting meal.

# Beet and Lentil Soup

## Ingredients:
- 1 tablespoon olive oil
- 1 onion, diced
- 2 carrots, diced
- 2 stalks celery, diced
- 3 cloves garlic, minced
- 1 cup dried green lentils, rinsed and drained
- 4 cups vegetable broth
- 2 medium beets, peeled and diced
- 1 teaspoon dried thyme
- Salt and pepper, to taste
- Greek yogurt (optional, for garnish)

## Procedure:
1. In a large pot, heat olive oil over medium heat. Add diced onion, carrots, and celery. Cook until vegetables are softened, about 5-7 minutes.
2. Add minced garlic to the pot and cook for another 2 minutes, stirring frequently.
3. Add dried green lentils, vegetable broth, diced beets, and dried thyme to the pot. Bring to a boil, then reduce heat and simmer for 25-30 minutes, until lentils and beets are tender.
4. Season with salt and pepper to taste. Serve hot, garnished with a dollop of Greek yogurt if desired.

Beet and Lentil Soup is a hearty and colorful dish that's perfect for supporting inflammation management. Beets are rich in betalains, which have anti-inflammatory and antioxidant properties, while lentils provide protein and fiber. Enjoy a bowl of this soup for a nourishing and satisfying meal.

## Spicy Black Bean Soup

**Ingredients:**

- 1 tablespoon olive oil
- 1 onion, diced
- 2 cloves garlic, minced
- 1 jalapeño pepper, seeded and diced
- 2 teaspoons ground cumin
- 1 teaspoon chili powder
- 2 cans (15 ounces each) black beans, drained and rinsed
- 4 cups vegetable broth
- 1 cup corn kernels (fresh or frozen)
- 1 (14.5-ounce) can diced tomatoes
- Salt and pepper, to taste
- Fresh cilantro (optional, for garnish)
- Avocado slices (optional, for garnish)

**Procedure:**

1. In a large pot, heat olive oil over medium heat. Add diced onion and cook until softened, about 5 minutes.
2. Add minced garlic and diced jalapeño pepper to the pot. Cook for another 2 minutes, stirring frequently.

3. Stir in ground cumin and chili powder, and cook for an additional minute.
4. Add black beans, vegetable broth, corn kernels, and diced tomatoes to the pot. Bring to a boil, then reduce heat and simmer for 20-25 minutes.
5. Use an immersion blender to puree a portion of the soup, leaving some beans and vegetables whole for texture.
6. Season with salt and pepper to taste. Serve hot, garnished with fresh cilantro and avocado slices if desired.

Spicy Black Bean Soup is a flavorful and satisfying dish that's perfect for supporting inflammation management. Black beans are rich in protein and fiber, while jalapeño peppers add a spicy kick and help boost metabolism. Enjoy a bowl of this soup for a nourishing and comforting meal.

## Conclusion

Incorporating anti-inflammatory soups into your diet can be a delicious and effective way to support inflammation management and promote overall health. From hearty vegetable stews to creamy pureed soups, there's a wide variety of flavors and textures to explore.

By focusing on nutrient-dense ingredients like vegetables, legumes, herbs, and spices, you can create soups that not only taste delicious but also provide your body with the essential nutrients it needs to thrive. Experiment with different combinations of ingredients and spices to find the flavors that you enjoy most.

Remember to listen to your body and choose soups that make you feel nourished and satisfied. With these 15 anti-inflammatory soup recipes in your repertoire, you'll be well-equipped to support your health and well-being one delicious bowl at a time.

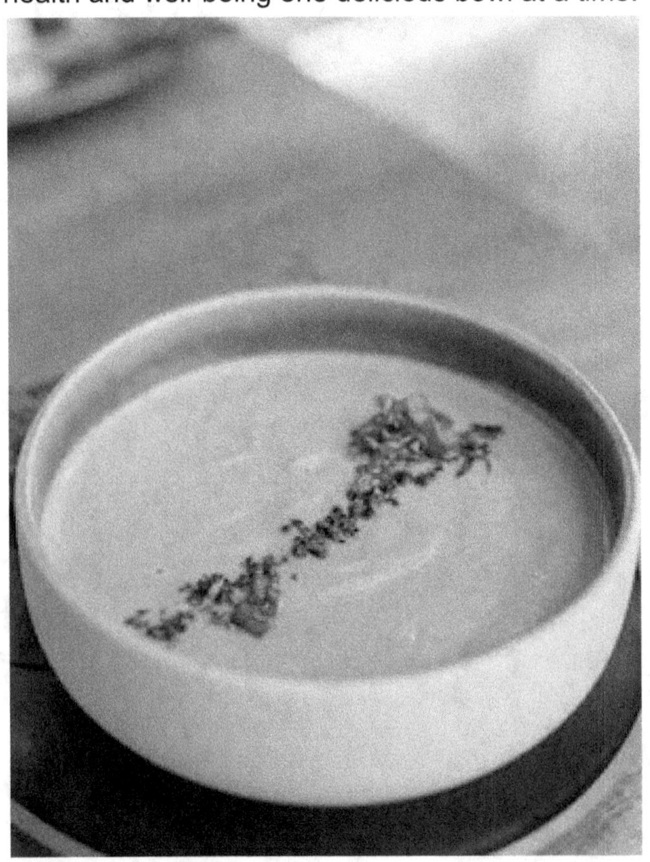

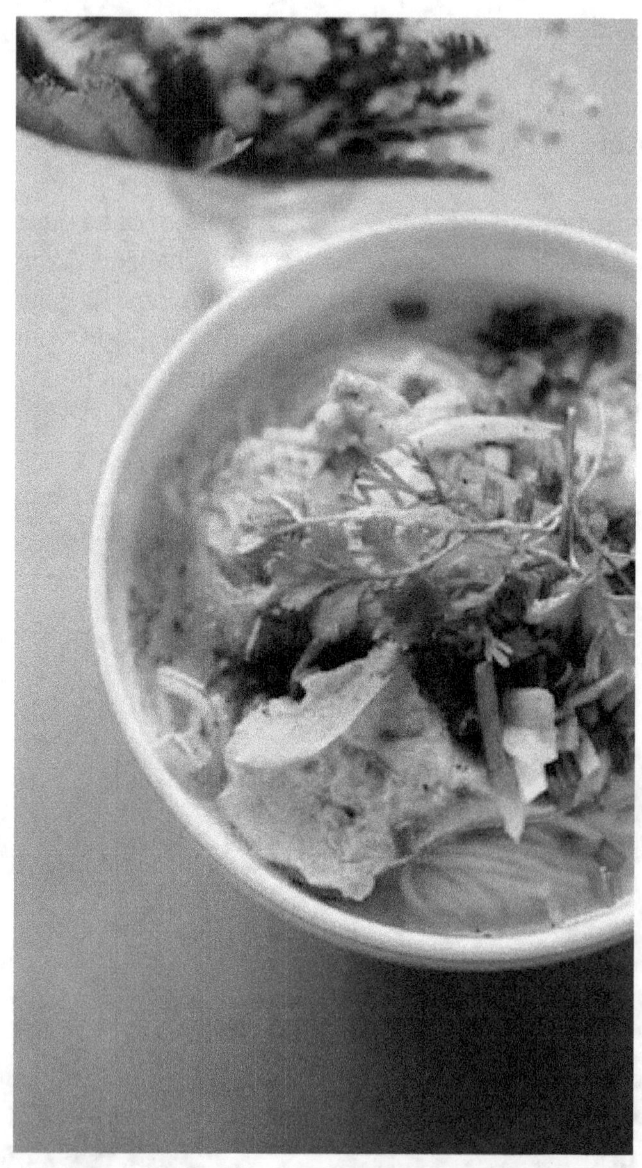

# CHAPTER FIVE

## Salads

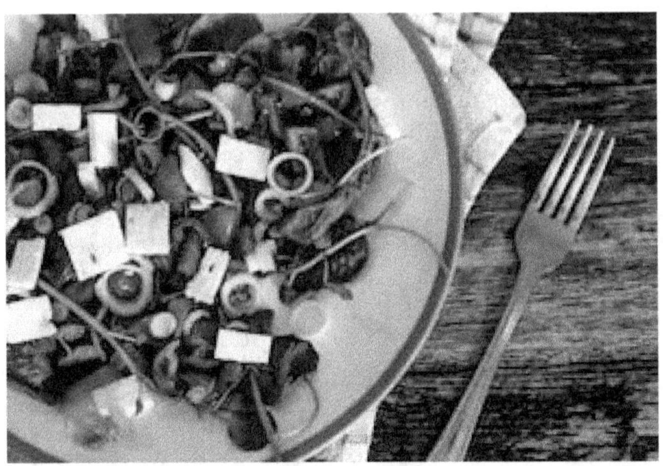

Inflammation, the body's natural response to injury or infection as we've explored, can wreak havoc if left unchecked. However, your diet can play a pivotal role in managing inflammation, and one delicious way to do so is by incorporating nutrient-rich salads into your meals. In this chapter, we'll explore 15 diverse salad recipes tailored specifically to combat inflammation while tantalizing your taste buds.

## Why Salads?

Before we dive into the delightful array of salad recipes, let's briefly touch on why salads are a stellar choice for battling inflammation. Packed with a plethora of vitamins, minerals, antioxidants, and phytonutrients, salads offer a potent blend of nutrients that help quell inflammation and promote overall wellness.

According to Dr. Amanda Hughes, a renowned nutritionist with over a decade of experience, "Salads are a powerhouse of anti-inflammatory compounds. Ingredients like leafy greens, colorful vegetables, nuts, seeds, and healthy fats work synergistically to dampen inflammation and support optimal health."

By incorporating a variety of ingredients known for their anti-inflammatory properties, salads become not only a delicious culinary delight but also a potent weapon in your arsenal against inflammation.

## Mediterranean Chickpea Salad

**Ingredients:**
- 1 can (15 ounces) chickpeas, drained and rinsed
- 1 cup cherry tomatoes, halved

- 1 cucumber, diced
- 1/4 cup red onion, finely chopped
- 1/4 cup Kalamata olives, pitted and sliced
- 2 tablespoons fresh parsley, chopped
- 2 tablespoons extra virgin olive oil
- 1 tablespoon lemon juice
- Salt and pepper to taste

**Procedure:**

1. In a large bowl, combine chickpeas, cherry tomatoes, cucumber, red onion, olives, and parsley.
2. Drizzle olive oil and lemon juice over the salad.
3. Season with salt and pepper, then toss to combine.
4. Serve chilled or at room temperature.

This Mediterranean Chickpea Salad is packed with fiber, antioxidants, and anti-inflammatory compounds. Chickpeas provide plant-based protein, while olive oil offers heart-healthy fats. The colorful array of vegetables adds vitamins and minerals, making this salad an excellent choice for fighting inflammation.

# Kale and Quinoa Salad (with Lemon Tahini Dressing)

**Ingredients:**

- 2 cups kale, chopped
- 1 cup cooked quinoa

- 1/4 cup almonds, chopped
- 1/4 cup dried cranberries
- 1/4 cup feta cheese, crumbled
- 2 tablespoons tahini
- 2 tablespoons lemon juice
- 1 tablespoon olive oil
- 1 clove garlic, minced
- Salt and pepper to taste

## Procedure:

1. In a large bowl, massage kale with olive oil until softened.
2. Add cooked quinoa, almonds, dried cranberries, and feta cheese to the bowl.
3. In a small bowl, whisk together tahini, lemon juice, olive oil, garlic, salt, and pepper to make the dressing.
4. Pour the dressing over the salad and toss to combine.
5. Serve immediately or refrigerate until ready to eat.

This salad is a nutritional powerhouse, with kale providing vitamins K, A, and C, while quinoa offers protein and fiber. The lemon tahini dressing adds a burst of flavor and healthy fats, making this salad an excellent choice for reducing inflammation and promoting overall well-being.

# Beet and Arugula Salad with Goat Cheese

## Ingredients:

- 2 medium beets, roasted and diced
- 4 cups arugula
- 1/4 cup walnuts, chopped
- 1/4 cup goat cheese, crumbled
- 2 tablespoons balsamic vinegar
- 1 tablespoon extra virgin olive oil
- Salt and pepper to taste

## Procedure:

1. In a large bowl, combine roasted beets, arugula, walnuts, and goat cheese.
2. Drizzle balsamic vinegar and olive oil over the salad.
3. Season with salt and pepper, then toss gently to combine.
4. Serve immediately.

Beets are rich in betalains, compounds known for their anti-inflammatory properties, while arugula provides a peppery flavor and vitamin K. The walnuts add omega-3 fatty acids, and goat cheese offers a creamy texture, making this salad a flavorful and nutritious choice for combating inflammation.

# Spinach and Strawberry Salad with Almonds

**Ingredients:**

- 4 cups baby spinach
- 1 cup strawberries, sliced
- 1/4 cup almonds, sliced
- 1/4 cup feta cheese, crumbled
- 2 tablespoons balsamic vinegar
- 1 tablespoon extra virgin olive oil
- 1 teaspoon honey (optional)
- Salt and pepper to taste

**Procedure:**

1. In a large bowl, combine baby spinach, sliced strawberries, almonds, and feta cheese.
2. In a small bowl, whisk together balsamic vinegar, olive oil, honey (if using), salt, and pepper to make the dressing.
3. Drizzle the dressing over the salad and toss gently to combine.
4. Serve immediately.

Spinach is loaded with vitamins and minerals, including vitamins A and C, which have anti-inflammatory properties. Strawberries provide antioxidants, while almonds offer heart-healthy fats. Combined with the tangy balsamic dressing, this salad is a delicious way to reduce inflammation.

# Grilled Veggie Quinoa Salad

**Ingredients:**

- 1 cup cooked quinoa
- 1 zucchini, sliced
- 1 yellow squash, sliced
- 1 red bell pepper, sliced
- 1 red onion, sliced
- 2 tablespoons extra virgin olive oil
- 2 tablespoons balsamic vinegar
- 1 teaspoon dried Italian herbs
- Salt and pepper to taste

**Procedure:**

1. Preheat grill to medium-high heat.
2. In a large bowl, toss sliced zucchini, yellow squash, red bell pepper, and red onion with olive oil, balsamic vinegar, Italian herbs, salt, and pepper.
3. Grill vegetables until tender and slightly charred, about 5-7 minutes per side.
4. In a large bowl, combine cooked quinoa with grilled vegetables.
5. Serve warm or at room temperature.

Grilled vegetables are rich in antioxidants, which help combat inflammation in the body. Quinoa adds protein and fiber, while the balsamic dressing provides flavor without excess calories. Enjoy this colorful and satisfying salad as a nutritious addition to your anti-inflammatory diet.

# Avocado and Black Bean Salad

## Ingredients:
- 1 can (15 ounces) black beans, drained and rinsed
- 1 avocado, diced
- 1 cup cherry tomatoes, halved
- 1/4 cup red onion, finely chopped
- 1/4 cup cilantro, chopped
- 2 tablespoons lime juice
- 1 tablespoon extra virgin olive oil
- Salt and pepper to taste

## Procedure:
1. In a large bowl, combine black beans, diced avocado, cherry tomatoes, red onion, and cilantro.
2. Drizzle lime juice and olive oil over the salad.
3. Season with salt and pepper, then toss gently to combine.
4. Serve chilled or at room temperature.

This recipe is loaded with fiber, healthy fats, and vitamins. Black beans provide plant-based protein, while avocado offers monounsaturated fats, which have anti-inflammatory properties. Enjoy this refreshing and satisfying salad as a delicious way to combat inflammation.

# Arugula, Pear, and Walnut Salad

**Ingredients:**

- 4 cups arugula
- 2 ripe pears, thinly sliced
- 1/4 cup walnuts, chopped
- 1/4 cup crumbled blue cheese
- 2 tablespoons apple cider vinegar
- 1 tablespoon extra virgin olive oil
- 1 teaspoon honey
- Salt and pepper to taste

**Procedure:**

1. In a large bowl, combine arugula, sliced pears, walnuts, and crumbled blue cheese.
2. In a small bowl, whisk together apple cider vinegar, olive oil, honey, salt, and pepper to make the dressing.
3. Drizzle the dressing over the salad and toss gently to combine.
4. Serve immediately.

This meal is bursting with flavor and nutrition. Arugula provides a peppery bite and vitamin K, while pears offer fiber and antioxidants. Walnuts add omega-3 fatty acids, and blue cheese contributes a creamy texture, making this salad a delightful choice for reducing inflammation.

# Asian-Inspired Cabbage Salad

## Ingredients:

- 4 cups shredded cabbage (green or purple)
- 1 cup shredded carrots
- 1/4 cup edamame, shelled
- 1/4 cup sliced almonds
- 2 green onions, thinly sliced
- 2 tablespoons rice vinegar
- 1 tablespoon low-sodium soy sauce
- 1 tablespoon sesame oil
- 1 teaspoon honey (optional)
- 1 teaspoon grated ginger
- Sesame seeds for garnish
- Salt and pepper to taste

## Procedure:

1. In a large bowl, combine shredded cabbage, shredded carrots, edamame, sliced almonds, and green onions.
2. In a small bowl, whisk together rice vinegar, soy sauce, sesame oil, honey (if using), grated ginger, salt, and pepper to make the dressing.
3. Drizzle the dressing over the salad and toss gently to combine.
4. Sprinkle sesame seeds on top for garnish.
5. Serve immediately.

This dish is a refreshing and crunchy one with a tangy dressing. Cabbage and carrots are rich in antioxidants and fiber, while edamame adds plant-based protein. The sesame oil and ginger contribute flavor and anti-inflammatory properties, making this salad a delicious choice for promoting overall health and well-being.

## Citrus and Avocado Salad

### Ingredients:
- 4 cups mixed greens (spinach, arugula, kale)
- 1 orange, peeled and segmented
- 1 grapefruit, peeled and segmented
- 1 avocado, diced
- 1/4 cup sliced almonds
- 2 tablespoons extra virgin olive oil
- 1 tablespoon apple cider vinegar
- 1 teaspoon honey
- Salt and pepper to taste

### Procedure:
1. In a large bowl, combine mixed greens, orange segments, grapefruit segments, diced avocado, and sliced almonds.
2. In a small bowl, whisk together olive oil, apple cider vinegar, honey, salt, and pepper to make the dressing.
3. Drizzle the dressing over the salad and toss gently to combine.
4. Serve immediately.

This meal is packed with flavor and nutrition. Oranges and grapefruits are rich in vitamin C and antioxidants, while avocado provides healthy fats and fiber. The combination of citrus and avocado creates a refreshing and satisfying salad that helps combat inflammation.

## Lentil and Vegetable Salad

### Ingredients:

- 1 cup cooked lentils
- 1 cup cherry tomatoes, halved
- 1 cucumber, diced
- 1/4 cup red onion, finely chopped
- 1/4 cup fresh parsley, chopped
- 2 tablespoons extra virgin olive oil
- 1 tablespoon balsamic vinegar
- 1 teaspoon Dijon mustard
- Salt and pepper to taste

### Procedure:

1. In a large bowl, combine cooked lentils, cherry tomatoes, cucumber, red onion, and parsley.
2. In a small bowl, whisk together olive oil, balsamic vinegar, Dijon mustard, salt, and pepper to make the dressing.
3. Drizzle the dressing over the salad and toss gently to combine.
4. Serve chilled or at room temperature.

This Lentil and Vegetable Salad is a nutritious and satisfying dish packed with plant-based protein, fiber, and antioxidants. Lentils provide a hearty base, while cherry tomatoes, cucumber, and red onion add freshness and flavor. Enjoy this salad as a delicious way to support a healthy inflammatory response.

# Broccoli and Chickpea Salad with Turmeric Dressing

## Ingredients:
- 2 cups broccoli florets, blanched
- 1 can (15 ounces) chickpeas, drained and rinsed
- 1/4 cup red onion, finely chopped
- 1/4 cup raisins
- 1/4 cup sliced almonds
- 2 tablespoons apple cider vinegar
- 1 tablespoon extra virgin olive oil
- 1 teaspoon ground turmeric
- 1 teaspoon honey
- Salt and pepper to taste

## Procedure:
1. In a large bowl, combine blanched broccoli florets, chickpeas, red onion, raisins, and sliced almonds.
2. In a small bowl, whisk together apple cider vinegar, olive oil, ground turmeric, honey, salt, and pepper to make the dressing.

3. Drizzle the dressing over the salad and toss gently to combine.
4. Serve chilled or at room temperature.

Broccoli is rich in antioxidants, while chickpeas provide protein and fiber. The turmeric dressing adds anti-inflammatory properties, making this salad a delicious choice for promoting overall health and well-being.

# Mixed Berry Spinach Salad (with Poppy Seed Dressing)

## Ingredients:
- 4 cups baby spinach
- 1 cup mixed berries (strawberries, blueberries, raspberries)
- 1/4 cup sliced almonds
- 1/4 cup feta cheese, crumbled
- 2 tablespoons balsamic vinegar
- 1 tablespoon extra virgin olive oil
- 1 teaspoon honey
- 1 teaspoon poppy seeds
- Salt and pepper to taste

## Procedure:
1. In a large bowl, combine baby spinach, mixed berries, sliced almonds, and crumbled feta cheese.

2. In a small bowl, whisk together balsamic vinegar, olive oil, honey, poppy seeds, salt, and pepper to make the dressing.
3. Drizzle the dressing over the salad and toss gently to combine.
4. Serve immediately.

This recipe is a delightful combination of sweet and savory flavors. Spinach provides vitamins and minerals, while mixed berries offer antioxidants. The poppy seed dressing adds a burst of flavor, making this salad a delicious choice for reducing inflammation and supporting overall well-being.

## Conclusion

In summary, anti-inflammatory salads offer a delicious and effective way to combat inflammation and promote overall health. Each salad recipe presented in this chapter is carefully crafted with nutrient-rich ingredients chosen for their ability to support a healthy inflammatory response. From Mediterranean-inspired creations to refreshing citrus combinations and hearty grain-based options, these salads provide a diverse range of flavors and textures to suit every palate. By incorporating colorful vegetables, leafy greens, lean proteins, healthy fats, and antioxidant-rich ingredients into your meals, you can nourish your body and reduce inflammation naturally. So, whether enjoyed as a light lunch, a side dish, or a satisfying main course, these salads are sure to delight your taste buds while supporting your well-being.

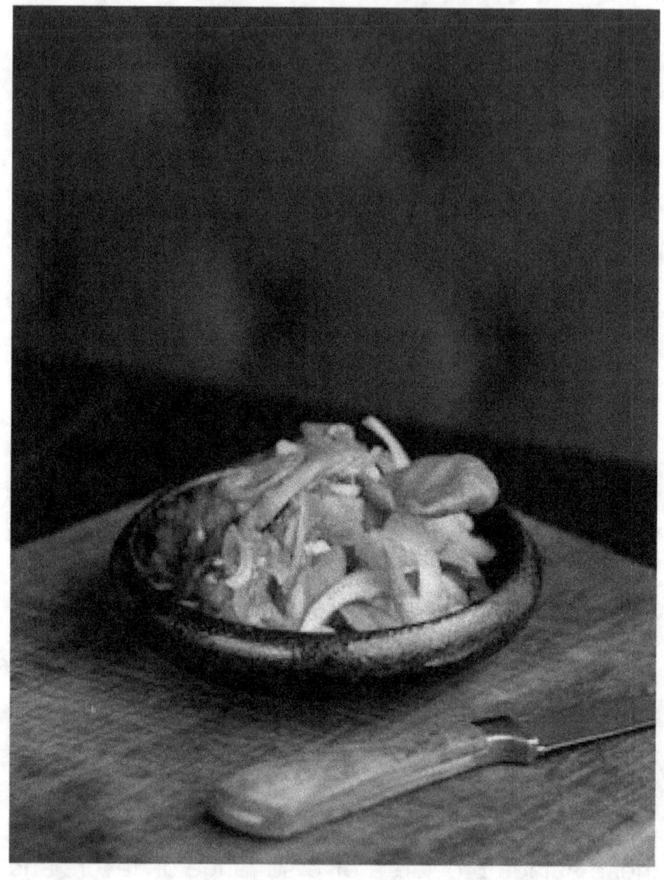

# CHAPTER SIX

## Pasta dishes

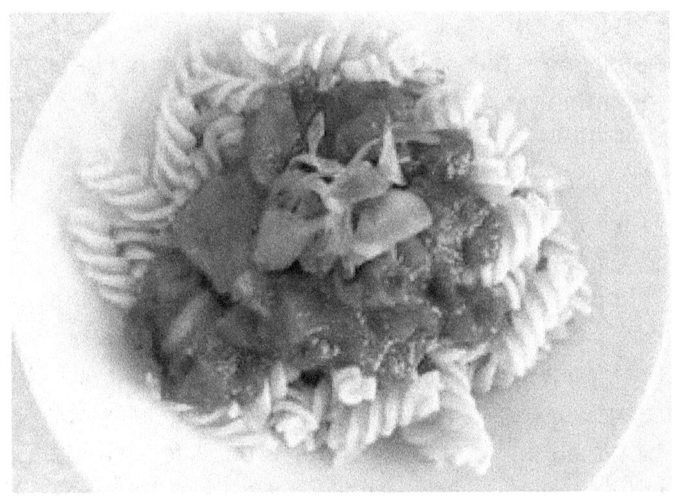

In the battle against inflammation, the kitchen can be your greatest ally as I keep emphasizing. While some may think that pasta dishes are off-limits for those seeking relief from inflammation, the truth is quite the opposite. When prepared with the right ingredients and techniques, pasta dishes can be both delicious and beneficial for reducing inflammation in the body.

# Why Pasta?

Pasta, a staple in many households, offers a versatile canvas for creating meals that are not only satisfying but also supportive of a healthy inflammatory response. The key lies in selecting the right type of pasta and pairing it with nutrient-rich ingredients that possess anti-inflammatory properties.

Whole grain pasta, such as whole wheat or brown rice pasta, is an excellent choice due to its higher fiber content and lower glycemic index compared to refined pasta. This means it can help stabilize blood sugar levels, which is crucial for managing inflammation. Additionally, whole grain pasta contains essential nutrients like vitamins, minerals, and antioxidants, which play a role in combating inflammation and promoting overall health.

Now, let's delve into 15 delectable pasta dishes designed to nourish your body and soothe inflammation. Each recipe is carefully crafted with ingredients known for their anti-inflammatory properties, making them not only delicious but also supportive of your health goals.

# Mediterranean Pasta Salad

## Ingredients:

- 8 ounces whole grain penne pasta
- 1 cup cherry tomatoes, halved
- 1 cucumber, diced
- 1/4 cup Kalamata olives, pitted and sliced
- 1/4 cup red onion, finely chopped
- 1/4 cup feta cheese, crumbled
- 2 tablespoons extra virgin olive oil
- 2 tablespoons red wine vinegar
- teaspoon dried oregano
- Salt and black pepper to taste

## Procedure:

1. Cook pasta according to package instructions. Drain and rinse under cold water.
2. In a large bowl, combine cooked pasta, cherry tomatoes, cucumber, olives, red onion, and feta cheese.
3. In a small bowl, whisk together olive oil, red wine vinegar, dried oregano, salt, and black pepper.
4. Pour the dressing over the pasta salad and toss to combine.
5. Serve chilled or at room temperature.

This is a refreshing and flavorful dish that incorporates the vibrant flavors of the Mediterranean diet. Rich in vegetables, olive oil, and herbs, it provides an abundance of antioxidants and anti-inflammatory compounds to support your health journey.

# Spinach and Mushroom Whole Wheat Pasta

**Ingredients:**
- 8 ounces whole wheat spaghetti
- 2 cups baby spinach leaves
- 1 cup cremini mushrooms, sliced
- 2 cloves garlic, minced
- 2 tablespoons olive oil
- 1/4 cup grated Parmesan cheese
- Salt and black pepper to taste
- Crushed red pepper flakes (optional)

**Procedure:**
1. Cook pasta according to package instructions. Drain and set aside.
2. In a large skillet, heat olive oil over medium heat. Add minced garlic and cook until fragrant, about 1 minute.
3. Add sliced mushrooms to the skillet and cook until they begin to soften, about 5 minutes.
4. Add baby spinach leaves to the skillet and cook until wilted, about 2 minutes.

5. Add cooked pasta to the skillet and toss to combine with the vegetables.
6. Season with salt, black pepper, and crushed red pepper flakes if desired.
7. Sprinkle grated Parmesan cheese over the pasta and toss to coat.
8. Serve hot, garnished with additional Parmesan cheese if desired.

This offers a hearty and nutritious meal that's quick and easy to prepare. Packed with fiber, vitamins, and minerals from the whole wheat pasta and leafy greens, it's a delicious way to support your body's natural anti-inflammatory processes.

## Roasted Vegetable Pasta Primavera

**Ingredients:**
- 8 ounces whole grain fusilli pasta
- 2 cups mixed vegetables (such as bell peppers, zucchini, and carrots), diced
- 2 tablespoons olive oil
- 2 cloves garlic, minced
- 1 teaspoon Italian seasoning
- Salt and black pepper to taste
- 1/4 cup grated Parmesan cheese (optional)

**Procedure:**
1. Preheat the oven to 400°F (200°C).
2. Toss diced vegetables with olive oil, minced garlic, Italian seasoning, salt, and black pepper.

3. Spread the vegetables in a single layer on a baking sheet and roast for 20-25 minutes, or until tender and slightly caramelized.
4. Cook pasta according to package instructions. Drain and set aside.
5. In a large skillet, combine cooked pasta and roasted vegetables. Heat gently until warmed through.
6. Serve hot, sprinkled with grated Parmesan cheese if desired.

This recipe is saturated with color and flavor, offering a satisfying way to incorporate a variety of nutrient-rich vegetables into your meal. With its vibrant array of antioxidants and fiber, it's a delightful addition to any anti-inflammatory diet.

## Lemon Garlic Shrimp Linguine

### Ingredients:
- 8 ounces whole wheat linguine
- 1 pound large shrimp, peeled and deveined
- 3 cloves garlic, minced
- Zest and juice of 1 lemon
- 2 tablespoons olive oil
- 2 tablespoons chopped fresh parsley
- Salt and black pepper to taste
- Lemon slices for garnish

### Procedure:
1. Cook pasta according to package instructions. Drain and set aside.

2.  In a large skillet, heat olive oil over medium heat. Add minced garlic and cook until fragrant, about 1 minute.
3.  Add shrimp to the skillet and cook until pink and opaque, about 2-3 minutes per side.
4.  Stir in lemon zest and juice, chopped parsley, salt, and black pepper.
5.  Add cooked linguine to the skillet and toss to coat with the shrimp and sauce.
6.  Serve hot, garnished with lemon slices.

This is a zesty and satisfying dish that's rich in protein and flavor. With the fresh citrusy notes of lemon and the savory aroma of garlic, it's sure to become a favorite in your anti-inflammatory repertoire.

## Vegetarian Eggplant and Tomato Pasta

**Ingredients:**
- 8 ounces whole grain spaghetti
- 1 large eggplant, diced
- 2 cups cherry tomatoes, halved
- 3 cloves garlic, minced
- 2 tablespoons olive oil
- 1/4 cup chopped fresh basil
- Salt and black pepper to taste
- Grated Parmesan cheese for garnish (optional)

**Procedure:**

1. Cook pasta according to package instructions. Drain and set aside.
2. In a large skillet, heat olive oil over medium heat. Add minced garlic and cook until fragrant, about 1 minute.
3. Add diced eggplant to the skillet and cook until tender and golden brown, about 10 minutes.
4. Add cherry tomatoes to the skillet and cook until they begin to soften, about 5 minutes.
5. Stir in chopped fresh basil and season with salt and black pepper.
6. Add cooked spaghetti to the skillet and toss to combine with the vegetables.
7. Serve hot, garnished with grated Parmesan cheese if desired.

This pasta meal celebrates the vibrant flavors of summer with its colorful array of vegetables. Eggplant, rich in antioxidants, pairs beautifully with sweet cherry tomatoes and fragrant basil, offering a wholesome and satisfying meal for inflammation relief.

## Chicken and Broccoli Alfredo

**Ingredients:**

- 8 ounces whole wheat fettuccine
- 2 boneless, skinless chicken breasts, cut into bite-sized pieces
- 2 cups broccoli florets

- 2 cloves garlic, minced
- 1 cup low-fat milk
- 1/2 cup grated Parmesan cheese
- 2 tablespoons olive oil
- Salt and black pepper to taste

## Procedure:

1. Cook pasta according to package instructions. Drain and set aside.
2. In a large skillet, heat olive oil over medium heat. Add minced garlic and cook until fragrant, about 1 minute.
3. Add chicken pieces to the skillet and cook until browned and cooked through, about 5-7 minutes.
4. Add broccoli florets to the skillet and cook until tender-crisp, about 3-4 minutes.
5. Reduce heat to low and pour in low-fat milk. Stir in grated Parmesan cheese until smooth and creamy.
6. Add cooked fettuccine to the skillet and toss to coat with the Alfredo sauce.
7. Serve hot, seasoned with salt and black pepper.

This offers a comforting and protein-packed meal that's sure to satisfy. With its creamy texture and wholesome ingredients, it's a guilt-free indulgence that supports your body's anti-inflammatory efforts.

# Red Lentil Pasta with Tomato Sauce

**Ingredients:**

- 8 ounces red lentil pasta
- 2 cups tomato sauce (homemade or store-bought)
- 1 cup cherry tomatoes, halved
- 2 cloves garlic, minced
- 1 tablespoon olive oil
- 1/4 cup chopped fresh basil
- Salt and black pepper to taste

**Procedure:**

1. Cook red lentil pasta according to package instructions. Drain and set aside.
2. In a large skillet, heat olive oil over medium heat. Add minced garlic and cook until fragrant, about 1 minute.
3. Add cherry tomatoes to the skillet and cook until they begin to soften, about 5 minutes.
4. Pour in tomato sauce and simmer for 5-10 minutes, allowing the flavors to meld.
5. Stir in chopped fresh basil and season with salt and black pepper.
6. Add cooked red lentil pasta to the skillet and toss to coat with the tomato sauce.
7. Serve hot, garnished with additional basil leaves if desired.

This Red Lentil Pasta with Tomato Sauce offers a nutritious twist on a classic favorite. Made with protein-rich red lentil pasta and flavorful tomato sauce, it's a satisfying dish that nourishes your body while helping to combat inflammation.

## Sautéed Spinach and Garlic Pasta

### Ingredients:

- 8 ounces whole grain spaghetti
- 4 cups baby spinach leaves
- 4 cloves garlic, minced
- 2 tablespoons olive oil
- 1/4 cup grated Parmesan cheese
- Salt and black pepper to taste
- Lemon zest for garnish (optional)

### Procedure:

1. Cook pasta according to package instructions. Drain and set aside.
2. In a large skillet, heat olive oil over medium heat. Add minced garlic and cook until fragrant, about 1 minute.
3. Add baby spinach leaves to the skillet and cook until wilted, about 2-3 minutes.
4. Add cooked spaghetti to the skillet and toss to combine with the spinach and garlic.
5. Season with salt and black pepper to taste.
6. Serve hot hot, garnished with grated Parmesan cheese and a sprinkle of lemon zest if desired.

This is a simple yet flavorful dish that celebrates the vibrant taste of fresh spinach and aromatic garlic. With its minimal ingredients and quick preparation, it's a convenient option for busy weeknights while providing essential nutrients to support your body's anti-inflammatory defenses.

## Mushroom and Spinach Whole Wheat Rotini

### Ingredients:

- 8 ounces whole wheat rotini pasta
- 2 cups cremini mushrooms, sliced
- 4 cups baby spinach leaves
- 3 cloves garlic, minced
- 2 tablespoons olive oil
- 1/4 cup grated Parmesan cheese
- Salt and black pepper to taste

### Procedure:

1. Cook pasta according to package instructions. Drain and set aside.
2. In a large skillet, heat olive oil over medium heat. Add minced garlic and cook until fragrant, about 1 minute.
3. Add sliced cremini mushrooms to the skillet and cook until they begin to release their juices, about 5-7 minutes.
4. Add baby spinach leaves to the skillet and cook until wilted, about 2-3 minutes.
5. Add cooked rotini pasta to the skillet and toss to combine with the mushrooms and spinach.
6. Season with salt and black pepper to taste.

7. Serve hot, garnished with grated Parmesan cheese.

This offers a delightful combination of earthy mushrooms and vibrant spinach, tossed with whole wheat pasta for a wholesome meal. Packed with antioxidants and fiber, it's a nourishing choice that supports your body's natural defenses against inflammation.

# Turkey Bolognese with Spaghetti Squash

## Ingredients:
- 1 medium spaghetti squash
- 1 pound ground turkey
- 1 onion, diced
- 2 cloves garlic, minced
- 2 cups tomato sauce (homemade or store-bought)
- 1 teaspoon dried oregano
- Salt and black pepper to taste
- Fresh basil leaves for garnish (optional)

## Procedure:
1. Preheat the oven to 375°F (190°C).
2. Cut the spaghetti squash in half lengthwise and remove the seeds.
3. Place the squash halves, cut side down, on a baking sheet lined with parchment paper.

Bake for 30-40 minutes, or until the squash is tender and easily pierced with a fork.
4. Using a fork, scrape the flesh of the squash to create "spaghetti" strands. Set aside.
5. In a large skillet, cook ground turkey over medium heat until browned and cooked through.
6. Add diced onion and minced garlic to the skillet and cook until softened, about 5 minutes.
7. Stir in tomato sauce and dried oregano. Simmer for 10-15 minutes to allow the flavors to meld.
8. Season with salt and black pepper to taste.
9. Serve the turkey Bolognese over the cooked spaghetti squash "noodles."
10. Garnish with fresh basil leaves if desired.

This recipe offers a lighter twist on a classic Italian favorite. By swapping traditional pasta for spaghetti squash, you can enjoy all the flavors of Bolognese sauce while reducing your carbohydrate intake and supporting a healthy inflammatory response.

## Lemon Asparagus Pasta with Grilled Chicken

**Ingredients:**
- 8 ounces whole wheat spaghetti
- 2 boneless, skinless chicken breasts
- 1 bunch asparagus, trimmed and cut into bite-sized pieces

- Zest and juice of 1 lemon
- 3 cloves garlic, minced
- 2 tablespoons olive oil
- Salt and black pepper to taste
- Fresh parsley for garnish (optional)

## Procedure:

1. Cook pasta according to package instructions. Drain and set aside.
2. Preheat a grill or grill pan over medium-high heat.
3. Season chicken breasts with salt, black pepper, and a drizzle of olive oil. Grill for 5-6 minutes per side, or until cooked through. Let rest for 5 minutes before slicing.
4. In a large skillet, heat olive oil over medium heat. Add minced garlic and cook until fragrant, about 1 minute.
5. Add asparagus to the skillet and cook until tender-crisp, about 4-5 minutes.
6. Add cooked spaghetti to the skillet and toss to combine with the asparagus.
7. Stir in lemon zest and juice, and season with salt and black pepper to taste.
8. Serve hot, topped with sliced grilled chicken.
9. Garnish with fresh parsley if desired.

This is a light and refreshing dish that's perfect for springtime. With its vibrant flavors and nutrient-rich ingredients, it's a wholesome choice that supports your body's anti-inflammatory efforts.

# Quinoa Pasta with Roasted Cherry Tomatoes and Basil

## Ingredients:

- 8 ounces quinoa pasta
- 2 cups cherry tomatoes
- 3 cloves garlic, minced
- 2 tablespoons olive oil
- 1/4 cup chopped fresh basil
- Salt and black pepper to taste
- Grated Parmesan cheese for garnish (optional)

## Procedure:

1. Cook quinoa pasta according to package instructions. Drain and set aside.
2. Preheat the oven to 400°F (200°C).
3. Toss cherry tomatoes with olive oil, minced garlic, salt, and black pepper.
4. Spread the tomatoes in a single layer on a baking sheet and roast for 20-25 minutes, or until they begin to burst and caramelize.
5. In a large skillet, combine cooked pasta with roasted cherry tomatoes and chopped fresh basil.
6. Toss to combine and heat gently until warmed through.
7. Serve hot, garnished with grated Parmesan cheese if desired.

This offers a gluten-free alternative to traditional pasta while delivering a burst of flavor and color.

With the sweet-tart taste of roasted tomatoes and the aromatic freshness of basil, it's a delightful choice for inflammation relief.

## Zucchini Noodles with Pesto and Grilled Shrimp

### Ingredients:

- 2 medium zucchini, spiralized into noodles
- 1 pound large shrimp, peeled and deveined
- 1/4 cup basil pesto (homemade or store-bought)
- 2 tablespoons olive oil
- 2 cloves garlic, minced
- Salt and black pepper to taste
- Grated Parmesan cheese for garnish (optional)

### Procedure:

1. In a large skillet, heat olive oil over medium heat. Add minced garlic and cook until fragrant, about 1 minute.
2. Add shrimp to the skillet and cook until pink and opaque, about 2-3 minutes per side.
3. Remove the shrimp from the skillet and set aside.
4. Add spiralized zucchini noodles to the skillet and cook until tender-crisp, about 2-3 minutes.
5. Return the cooked shrimp to the skillet and toss with basil pesto until evenly coated.

6. Season with salt and black pepper to taste
7. Serve hot, garnished with grated Parmesan cheese.

This offers a low-carb alternative to traditional pasta, making it a perfect choice for those seeking to reduce inflammation while still enjoying delicious flavors. With the vibrant green of the zucchini noodles, the bold taste of basil pesto, and the succulent grilled shrimp, it's a satisfying dish that's as visually appealing as it is flavorful.

## Spaghetti Squash Carbonara

### Ingredients:
- 1 medium spaghetti squash
- 4 slices nitrate-free bacon, chopped
- 3 cloves garlic, minced
- 2 eggs
- 1/2 cup grated Parmesan cheese
- Salt and black pepper to taste
- Chopped fresh parsley for garnish (optional)

### Procedure:
1. Preheat the oven to 375°F (190°C).
2. Cut the spaghetti squash in half lengthwise and remove the seeds.
3. Place the squash halves, cut side down, on a baking sheet lined with parchment paper. Bake for 30-40 minutes, or until the squash is tender and easily pierced with a fork.

4. Using a fork, scrape the flesh of the squash to create "spaghetti" strands. Set aside.
5. In a large skillet, cook chopped bacon over medium heat until crispy. Remove bacon from the skillet and set aside, leaving the rendered fat in the skillet.
6. Add minced garlic to the skillet and cook until fragrant, about 1 minute.
7. In a small bowl, whisk together eggs and grated Parmesan cheese.
8. Add cooked spaghetti squash "noodles" to the skillet with the garlic and toss to coat with the bacon fat.
9. Remove the skillet from heat and quickly stir in the egg and cheese mixture, tossing to combine until the sauce thickens.
10. Season with salt and black pepper to taste.
11. Serve hot, garnished with chopped fresh parsley if desired.

This meal offers a lighter take on the classic Italian dish, replacing traditional pasta with spaghetti squash for a lower-carb, inflammation-fighting alternative. With its creamy texture, savory bacon, and hints of garlic and Parmesan cheese, it's a comforting and satisfying meal for any occasion.

# Vegetable Stir-Fry with Soba Noodles

## Ingredients:

- 8 ounces soba noodles
- 2 cups mixed vegetables (such as bell peppers, snap peas, and carrots), sliced
- 3 cloves garlic, minced
- 2 tablespoons low-sodium soy sauce
- 1 tablespoon sesame oil
- 1 tablespoon rice vinegar
- 1 teaspoon grated ginger
- Sesame seeds for garnish (optional)
- Sliced green onions for garnish (optional)

## Procedure:

1. Cook soba noodles according to package instructions. Drain and set aside.
2. In a large skillet or wok, heat sesame oil over medium-high heat. Add minced garlic and grated ginger and cook until fragrant, about 1 minute.
3. Add sliced mixed vegetables to the skillet and stir-fry until tender-crisp, about 3-5 minutes.
4. Add cooked soba noodles to the skillet, along with low-sodium soy sauce and rice vinegar.
5. Toss to combine and heat through.

6. Serve hot, garnished with sesame seeds and sliced green onions if desired.

This offers a nutrient-packed meal that's as colorful as it is delicious. With a medley of fresh vegetables, savory soy sauce, and fragrant ginger, it's a flavorful way to enjoy the benefits of anti-inflammatory ingredients while satisfying your cravings for a comforting noodle dish.

## Conclusion:

In conclusion, these 15 pasta dishes showcase the versatility and health benefits of incorporating pasta into an anti-inflammatory diet. From whole grain varieties packed with fiber and nutrients to innovative vegetable-based alternatives, there's a pasta dish to suit every taste and dietary preference. By choosing wholesome ingredients rich in antioxidants, vitamins, and minerals, you can nourish your body while enjoying delicious and satisfying meals that support your journey towards inflammation relief. So, don't hesitate to explore these recipes and discover the joys of pasta as a powerful ally in your quest for optimal health and well-being.

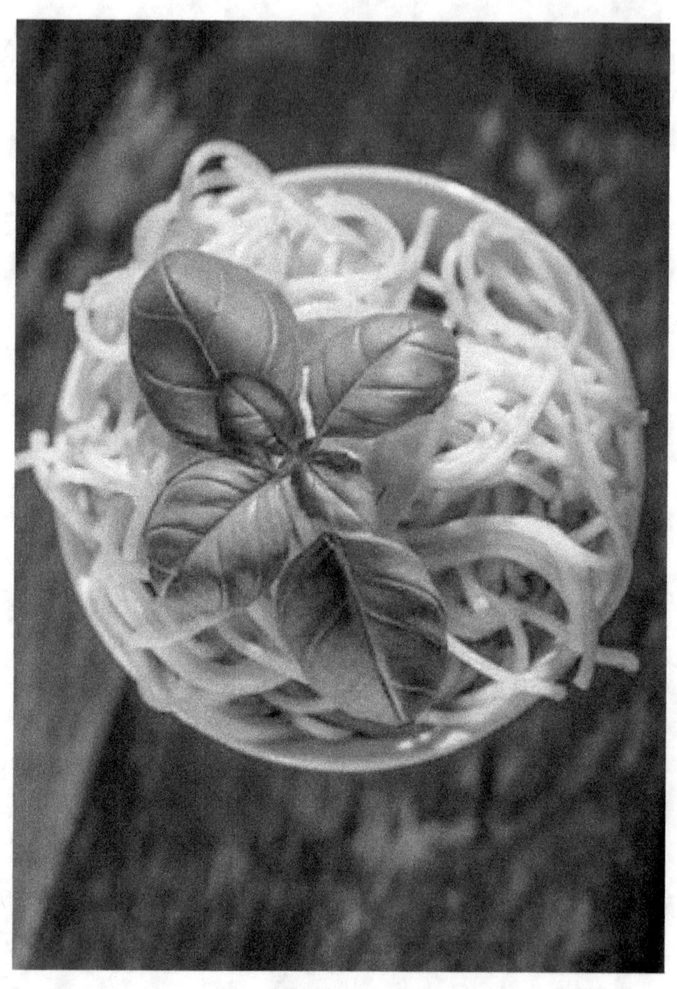

# CHAPTER SEVEN

## Sandwiches

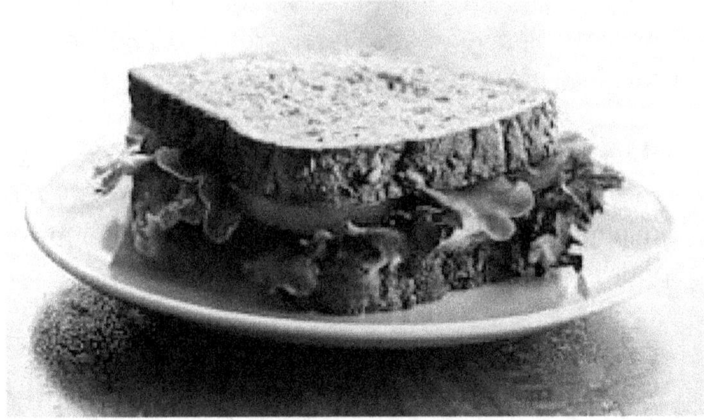

Sandwiches are not just convenient meals; they can also be powerful allies in the fight against inflammation. As you delve into the world of anti-inflammatory eating, incorporating sandwiches into your diet can offer both nourishment and flavor. In this chapter, we'll explore 15 delicious sandwich recipes designed specifically to combat inflammation and promote overall health.

## Why Sandwich?

Like pastas, sandwiches provide an excellent platform for incorporating a variety of anti-inflammatory ingredients. By carefully selecting the components of your sandwich, you can create a balanced meal that supports your body's natural healing processes.

In the words of Dr. Maria Rodriguez, "Sandwiches can be incredibly versatile and nutritious when prepared with inflammation-fighting ingredients such as leafy greens, lean proteins, and healthy fats."

Sandwiches are also very convenient. They're easy to prepare. An average sandwich takes 5 - 10 minutes, making them excellent choices for busy individuals.

Let's look at 15 sandwich recipes you should try, that fight against inflammation.

## Mediterranean Veggie Sandwich

**Ingredients:**
- 2 slices whole grain bread
- 2 tablespoons hummus
- 1/4 cup cucumber, thinly sliced
- 1/4 cup red bell pepper, thinly sliced
- 1/4 cup red onion, thinly sliced
- 1/4 cup mixed greens
- 2 tablespoons feta cheese, crumbled
- 1 tablespoon Kalamata olives, sliced
- 1 teaspoon olive oil
- Salt and pepper to taste

**Procedure:**

1. Spread hummus evenly on one slice of bread.
2. Layer cucumber, red bell pepper, red onion, and mixed greens on top of the hummus.
3. Sprinkle crumbled feta cheese and sliced Kalamata olives over the vegetables.
4. Drizzle olive oil over the filling and season with salt and pepper.
5. Top with the second slice of bread and press gently to hold the sandwich together.
6. Slice in half diagonally and serve.

The sandwich is dense with flavor and nutrients. Packed with colorful vegetables, creamy hummus, and tangy feta cheese, this sandwich offers a delightful combination of textures and tastes. The inclusion of olive oil provides a dose of healthy fats, while the Kalamata olives add a savory punch. Enjoy this sandwich as a satisfying meal that supports your body's anti-inflammatory efforts.

## Grilled Chicken and Avocado Wrap

### Ingredients:
- 1 whole wheat tortilla
- 3 ounces grilled chicken breast, sliced
- 1/4 avocado, sliced
- 1/4 cup baby spinach leaves
- 1 tablespoon Greek yogurt
- 1 teaspoon Dijon mustard
- Salt and pepper to taste

**Procedure:**

1. Lay the whole wheat tortilla flat on a clean surface.
2. Spread Greek yogurt and Dijon mustard evenly on the tortilla.
3. Layer grilled chicken slices, avocado slices, and baby spinach leaves on top.
4. Season with salt and pepper to taste.
5. Roll the tortilla tightly into a wrap.
6. Slice in half diagonally and serve.

This sandwich is a protein-packed option that combines grilled chicken breast with creamy avocado and crisp spinach. Greek yogurt adds creaminess without the need for mayonnaise, while Dijon mustard provides a tangy kick. Enjoy this satisfying wrap as a nutritious meal that helps combat inflammation.

## Turkey and Cranberry Panini

**Ingredients:**

- 2 slices whole grain bread
- 3 ounces sliced turkey breast
- 1 tablespoon cranberry sauce
- 1 tablespoon Dijon mustard
- 1/4 cup baby spinach leaves
- 1 slice provolone cheese
- 1 teaspoon olive oil

**Procedure:**

1. Spread Dijon mustard on one slice of whole grain bread.
2. Layer sliced turkey breast, cranberry sauce, baby spinach leaves, and provolone cheese on top.
3. Top with the second slice of bread.
4. Brush olive oil on the outside of the sandwich.
5. Place the sandwich in a panini press or grill pan and cook until the bread is toasted and the cheese is melted.
6. Slice in half diagonally and serve hot.

This offers a delightful blend of savory turkey, sweet cranberry sauce, and melty provolone cheese. With the added goodness of whole grain bread and fresh spinach, this sandwich is a flavorful way to incorporate anti-inflammatory ingredients into your diet.

## Veggie and Hummus Pita Pocket

### Ingredients:

- 1 whole wheat pita pocket, halved
- 2 tablespoons hummus
- 1/4 cup cucumber, diced
- 1/4 cup cherry tomatoes, halved
- 1/4 cup shredded carrots
- 1/4 cup mixed greens
- 1 tablespoon feta cheese, crumbled
- Lemon juice and olive oil for drizzling
- Salt and pepper to taste

**Procedure:**

1. Spread hummus inside each half of the pita pocket.
2. Fill with diced cucumber, cherry tomatoes, shredded carrots, mixed greens, and crumbled feta cheese.
3. Drizzle with lemon juice and olive oil.
4. Season with salt and pepper to taste.
5. Serve immediately.

This is a refreshing and nutrient-packed option that combines crunchy vegetables with creamy hummus. Packed into a convenient pita pocket, this sandwich is perfect for on-the-go lunches or quick and easy dinners. Enjoy the vibrant flavors and anti-inflammatory benefits of this delicious creation.

## Salmon and Avocado Bagel

**Ingredients:**

- 1 whole grain bagel, halved and toasted
- 3 ounces cooked salmon fillet
- 1/4 avocado, mashed
- 1 tablespoon Greek yogurt
- 1 teaspoon capers
- 1 tablespoon red onion, thinly sliced
- 1 tablespoon fresh dill, chopped
- Lemon wedges for serving
- Salt and pepper to taste

**Procedure:**

1. Spread mashed avocado on one half of the toasted bagel.
2. Mix Greek yogurt, capers, red onion, and fresh dill in a small bowl.
3. Spread the yogurt mixture on the other half of the bagel.
4. Layer cooked salmon fillet on top of the avocado.
5. Season with salt and pepper to taste.
6. Serve with lemon wedges on the side.

This bagel offers a delectable combination of omega-3-rich salmon, creamy avocado, and tangy yogurt sauce. With the added zing of capers and fresh dill, this sandwich is bursting with flavor and nutritional benefits. Enjoy this satisfying meal as a tasty way to support your body's anti-inflammatory efforts.

## Chickpea Salad Sandwich

**Ingredients:**

- 1/2 cup canned chickpeas, drained and rinsed
- 1 tablespoon Greek yogurt
- 1 tablespoon lemon juice
- 1/4 cup celery, finely chopped
- 1 tablespoon red onion, finely chopped
- 1 tablespoon fresh parsley, chopped
- Salt and pepper to taste
- 2 slices whole grain bread

- Lettuce leaves and tomato slices for serving

**Procedure:**
1. In a mixing bowl, mash the chickpeas with a fork until slightly chunky.
2. Stir in Greek yogurt, lemon juice, celery, red onion, and parsley until well combined.
3. Season with salt and pepper to taste.
4. Spread the chickpea mixture onto one slice of bread.
5. Top with lettuce leaves, tomato slices, and the second slice of bread.
6. Slice in half diagonally and serve.

This sandwich offers a plant-based alternative to traditional meat-filled sandwiches. Packed with protein and fiber from chickpeas, and freshness from vegetables, this sandwich is both satisfying and nutritious. Enjoy the delicious flavors and anti-inflammatory benefits of this simple yet flavorful creation.

## Egg and Spinach Breakfast Sandwich

**Ingredients:**
- 1 whole grain English muffin, halved and toasted
- 1 large egg
- 1/4 cup baby spinach leaves
- 1 slice tomato

- 1 slice avocado
- Salt and pepper to taste

**Procedure:**
1. Heat a non-stick skillet over medium heat.
2. Crack the egg into the skillet and cook to desired doneness.
3. Season with salt and pepper to taste.
4. Assemble the sandwich by layering baby spinach leaves, tomato slice, cooked egg, and avocado on one half of the toasted English muffin.
5. Top with the other half of the English muffin.
6. Serve immediately.

This is a nutritious and filling option to start your day on the right foot. With protein-rich egg, nutrient-packed spinach, and creamy avocado, this sandwich provides a satisfying and balanced breakfast. Enjoy the flavors and benefits of this delicious morning meal as you support your body's anti-inflammatory needs.

## Tofu Banh Mi Sandwich

**Ingredients:**
- 1 small baguette, cut in half lengthwise
- 4 ounces extra-firm tofu, sliced and pressed
- 2 tablespoons soy sauce
- 1 tablespoon rice vinegar
- 1 teaspoon sesame oil
- 1 teaspoon Sriracha sauce

- 1/4 cup shredded carrots
- 1/4 cup cucumber, thinly sliced
- 2 tablespoons fresh cilantro leaves
- 2 tablespoons mayonnaise
- 1 tablespoon hoisin sauce

**Procedure:**

1. In a bowl, whisk together soy sauce, rice vinegar, sesame oil, and Sriracha sauce.
2. Marinate tofu slices in the mixture for 15 minutes
3. Heat a skillet over medium heat and cook tofu slices until golden brown on each side.
4. Spread mayonnaise and hoisin sauce on one half of the baguette.
5. Layer cooked tofu slices, shredded carrots, cucumber slices, and fresh cilantro leaves on top.
6. Top with the other half of the baguette.
7. Slice into individual portions and serve.

This offers a vegetarian twist on the classic Vietnamese street food favorite. With marinated tofu, crunchy vegetables, and a flavorful sauce, this sandwich is a delicious and satisfying meal option. Enjoy the bold flavors and anti-inflammatory benefits of this tasty creation.

## Turkey and Apple Wrap

**Ingredients:**

- 1 whole wheat tortilla

- 3 ounces sliced turkey breast
- 1/4 apple, thinly sliced
- 1/4 cup mixed greens
- 1 tablespoon Greek yogurt
- 1 teaspoon honey
- 1/2 teaspoon Dijon mustard
- Salt and pepper to taste

**Procedure:**
1. Lay the whole wheat tortilla flat on a clean surface.
2. Spread Greek yogurt, honey, and Dijon mustard evenly on the tortilla.
3. Layer sliced turkey breast, apple slices, and mixed greens on top.
4. Season with salt and pepper to taste.
5. Roll the tortilla tightly into a wrap.
6. Slice in half diagonally and serve.

This offers a delightful combination of savory turkey, sweet apple, and tangy yogurt sauce. With the added freshness of mixed greens, this wrap provides a satisfying and nutritious meal option. Enjoy the flavors and anti-inflammatory benefits of this delicious creation.

## Caprese Panini

**Ingredients:**
- 2 slices whole grain bread
- 2 slices fresh mozzarella cheese
- 1/2 cup fresh basil leaves

- 1 small tomato, thinly sliced
- 1 teaspoon balsamic glaze
- Salt and pepper to taste
- Olive oil for brushing

## Procedure:

1. Layer fresh mozzarella cheese, basil leaves, and tomato slices on one slice of bread.
2. Drizzle balsamic glaze over the tomato slices.
3. Season with salt and pepper to taste.
4. Top with the second slice of bread.
5. Brush olive oil on the outside of the sandwich.
6. Place the sandwich in a panini press or grill pan and cook until the bread is toasted and the cheese is melted.
7. Slice in half diagonally and serve hot.

This iis a classic Italian-inspired sandwich featuring the timeless combination of fresh mozzarella, ripe tomatoes, and fragrant basil. With a drizzle of balsamic glaze adding sweetness and depth of flavor, this panini is a delicious and satisfying meal option. Enjoy the vibrant flavors and anti-inflammatory benefits of this delightful creation.

## Smoked Salmon Bagel Sandwich

### Ingredients:

- 1 whole grain bagel, halved and toasted

- 2 ounces smoked salmon
- 2 tablespoons cream cheese
- 1 tablespoon capers
- 1 tablespoon red onion, thinly sliced
- 1 tablespoon fresh dill, chopped
- Lemon wedges for serving
- Salt and pepper to taste

**Procedure:**

1. Spread cream cheese on one half of the toasted bagel.
2. Layer smoked salmon, capers, red onion, and fresh dill on top.
3. Squeeze lemon juice over the salmon.
4. Season with salt and pepper to taste.
5. Top with the other half of the bagel.
6. Serve with lemon wedges on the side.

This offers a luxurious combination of rich smoked salmon, creamy cream cheese, and zesty toppings. With the added brightness of capers, red onion, and fresh dill, this sandwich is a flavorful and satisfying meal option. Enjoy the indulgent flavors and anti-inflammatory benefits of this delicious creation.

# Mediterranean Tuna Salad Sandwich

**Ingredients:**

- 1 can (5 ounces) tuna, drained

- 2 tablespoons Greek yogurt
- 1 tablespoon lemon juice
- 1/4 cup cucumber, diced
- 1/4 cup cherry tomatoes, halved
- 2 tablespoons Kalamata olives, sliced
- 1 tablespoon red onion, finely chopped
- 1 tablespoon fresh parsley, chopped
- Salt and pepper to taste
- 2 slices whole grain bread
- Lettuce leaves for serving

## Procedure:

1. In a mixing bowl, combine tuna, Greek yogurt, lemon juice, cucumber, cherry tomatoes, Kalamata olives, red onion, and parsley.
2. Season with salt and pepper to taste.
3. Spread the tuna salad mixture onto one slice of bread.
4. Top with lettuce leaves and the second slice of bread.
5. Slice in half diagonally and serve.

This offers a burst of flavors inspired by the Mediterranean diet. With protein-rich tuna, refreshing vegetables, and tangy Greek yogurt, this sandwich is a nutritious and satisfying meal option. Enjoy the vibrant flavors and anti-inflammatory benefits of this delicious creation.

# Grilled Vegetable Panini

**Ingredients:**

- 2 slices whole grain bread
- 1/2 zucchini, thinly sliced lengthwise
- 1/2 yellow squash, thinly sliced lengthwise
- 1/4 red bell pepper, thinly sliced
- 1/4 yellow bell pepper, thinly sliced
- 1/4 red onion, thinly sliced
- 2 tablespoons pesto sauce
- 1 slice provolone cheese
- Olive oil for brushing

**Procedure:**

1. Preheat a grill pan over medium heat.
2. Brush olive oil on both sides of the sliced vegetables.
3. Grill the vegetables until tender and lightly charred, about 2-3 minutes per side.
4. Spread pesto sauce on one slice of bread.
5. Layer grilled vegetables and provolone cheese on top.
6. Top with the second slice of bread.
7. Brush olive oil on the outside of the sandwich.
8. Place the sandwich in a panini press or grill pan and cook until the bread is toasted and the cheese is melted.
9. Slice in half diagonally and serve hot.

This is a celebration of colorful vegetables and bold flavors. With tender grilled zucchini, squash, peppers, and onions, layered with creamy pesto sauce and melty provolone cheese, this sandwich is a satisfying and nutritious meal option. Enjoy the delicious flavors and anti-inflammatory benefits of this delightful creation.

# Hummus and Roasted Red Pepper Wrap

## Ingredients:
- 1 whole wheat tortilla
- 2 tablespoons hummus
- 1/4 cup roasted red peppers, sliced
- 1/4 cup baby spinach leaves
- 1 tablespoon feta cheese, crumbled
- 1 tablespoon fresh parsley, chopped
- Lemon juice for drizzling
- Salt and pepper to taste

## Procedure:
1. Spread hummus evenly on the whole wheat tortilla.
2. Layer roasted red peppers, baby spinach leaves, crumbled feta cheese, and chopped parsley on top.
3. Drizzle with lemon juice.
4. Season with salt and pepper to taste.
5. Roll the tortilla tightly into a wrap.
6. Slice in half diagonally and serve.

With creamy hummus, sweet roasted red peppers, and tangy feta cheese, this wrap offers a delightful combination of flavors and textures. Enjoy the deliciousness and anti-inflammatory benefits of this simple yet satisfying creation.

## Avocado and Black Bean Quesadilla

Ingredients:
- 2 whole grain tortillas
- 1/2 avocado, mashed
- 1/4 cup black beans, cooked and mashed
- 2 tablespoons salsa
- 2 tablespoons shredded cheddar cheese
- Fresh cilantro leaves for garnish
- Lime wedges for serving
- Salt and pepper to taste

**Procedure:**
1. Spread mashed avocado on one tortilla.
2. Spread mashed black beans on the other tortilla.
3. Layer salsa and shredded cheddar cheese on top of the black beans.
4. Place the avocado-topped tortilla on top of the cheese-topped tortilla to form a sandwich.
5. Heat a non-stick skillet over medium heat.
6. Place the quesadilla in the skillet and cook until golden brown and crispy on both sides, about 2-3 minutes per side.

7. Slice into wedges and serve with fresh cilantro leaves and lime wedges on the side.

This is a tasty and nutritious twist on the classic Mexican dish. With creamy avocado, protein-packed black beans, zesty salsa, and melty cheddar cheese, this quesadilla offers a satisfying meal option. Enjoy the flavors and anti-inflammatory benefits of this delicious creation.

## Conclusion

In this chapter, we've introduced 15 nutritious sandwich recipes tailored to support an anti-inflammatory diet. From Mediterranean-inspired wraps to protein-packed paninis and savory quesadillas, each recipe offers a flavorful combination of ingredients chosen for their anti-inflammatory properties. By incorporating whole grains, lean proteins, healthy fats, and vibrant vegetables, these sandwiches provide a balanced and delicious way to combat inflammation and promote overall health. With options ranging from the Turkey and Apple Wrap to the Grilled Vegetable Panini and the Avocado and Black Bean Quesadilla, there's something to satisfy every craving while nourishing your body with ingredients that support optimal wellness. Enjoy exploring these flavorful creations and embrace the journey to a healthier lifestyle through the power of delicious, inflammation-fighting sandwiches.

# CHAPTER EIGHT

## Stir-fries

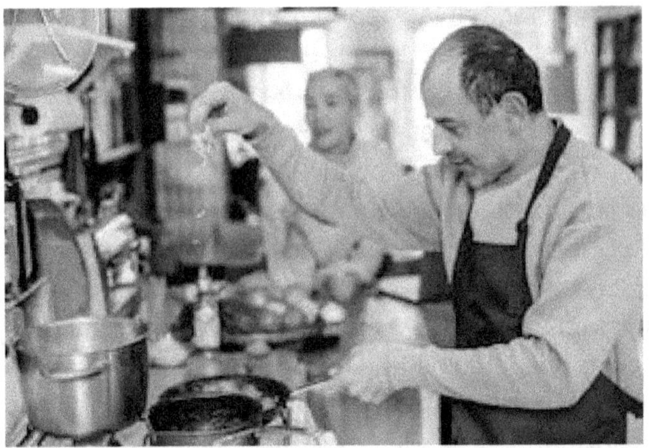

Stir fry dishes have long been celebrated not just for their delicious flavors but also for their health benefits. Whether you're a seasoned chef or a novice in the kitchen, stir fries offer a versatile canvas for creating nutritious and inflammation-fighting meals. As we delve into the art of stir frying, you'll discover how to prepare 15 delectable dishes designed to nourish your body and combat inflammation.

# Why Stir Fries?

Stir fries are a culinary wonder, combining a vibrant array of vegetables, lean proteins, and wholesome grains, all cooked to perfection in a sizzling pan. What makes stir fries particularly appealing for those seeking relief from inflammation is their emphasis on fresh, whole ingredients. As we saw in earlier chapters and I emphasize here again, fresh fruits and vegetables are laced with an abundance of nutrients which are arsenals against inflammation. By incorporating an abundance of colorful vegetables and lean proteins, stir fry dishes pack a powerful punch of vitamins, minerals, and antioxidants – all essential components for promoting optimal health and reducing inflammation in the body.

In short, stir fry dishes offer a delicious and convenient way to nourish your body while combating inflammation. By embracing the art of stir frying and incorporating nutrient-rich ingredients into your meals, you can enjoy a diverse array of flavors while supporting your overall health and well-being. In the following sections, we'll explore 15 tantalizing stir fry recipes designed to tantalize your taste buds and promote inflammation relief. So grab your apron and let's get cooking

# Veggie-Packed Chicken Stir Fry

## Ingredients:

- 1 lb boneless, skinless chicken breast, thinly sliced
- 2 cups mixed vegetables (bell peppers, broccoli, carrots, snap peas)
- 2 cloves garlic, minced
- 1 tablespoon fresh ginger, grated
- 2 tablespoons low-sodium soy sauce
- 1 tablespoon rice vinegar
- 1 teaspoon sesame oil
- 1 tablespoon olive oil
- Salt and pepper to taste
- Cooked brown rice or quinoa for serving

## Procedure:

1. In a large skillet or wok, heat olive oil over medium-high heat.
2. Add chicken and cook until browned and cooked through, about 5-6 minutes. Remove from skillet and set aside.
3. In the same skillet, add a bit more olive oil if needed. Add garlic and ginger, and cook for 1-2 minutes until fragrant.
4. Add mixed vegetables to the skillet and stir fry until crisp-tender, about 3-4 minutes.
5. Return cooked chicken to the skillet. Add soy sauce, rice vinegar, and sesame oil. Stir well to combine and coat the ingredients evenly.

6. Cook for an additional 2-3 minutes, until the sauce has thickened slightly and everything is heated through.
7. Serve hot over cooked brown rice or quinoa.

This is a perfect example of how stir fries can be both nutritious and delicious. Packed with lean protein, colorful vegetables, and aromatic spices, this dish provides a satisfying meal that can help alleviate inflammation and support overall health. Plus, it's quick and easy to prepare, making it ideal for busy weeknights. Enjoy the flavors and reap the benefits of this inflammation-fighting stir fry!

## Shrimp and Asparagus Stir Fry

**Ingredients:**
- 1 lb large shrimp, peeled and deveined
- 1 bunch asparagus, trimmed and cut into bite-sized pieces
- 2 cloves garlic, minced
- 1 tablespoon fresh ginger, grated
- 2 tablespoons low-sodium soy sauce
- 1 tablespoon honey or maple syrup
- 1 tablespoon rice vinegar
- 1 teaspoon sesame oil
- 1 tablespoon olive oil
- Salt and pepper to taste
- Cooked brown rice or quinoa for serving

**Procedure:**

1. Heat olive oil in a large skillet or wok over medium-high heat. Add garlic and ginger, and cook for 1-2 minutes until fragrant.
2. Add shrimp to the skillet and cook until pink and opaque, about 2-3 minutes per side. Remove shrimp from skillet and set aside.
3. In the same skillet, add a bit more olive oil if needed. Add asparagus and stir fry until tender-crisp, about 3-4 minutes.
4. Return cooked shrimp to the skillet. Add soy sauce, honey or maple syrup, rice vinegar, and sesame oil. Stir well to combine and coat the ingredients evenly.
5. Cook for an additional 2-3 minutes, until the sauce has thickened slightly and everything is heated through.
6. Serve hot over cooked brown rice or quinoa.

This shrimp and asparagus stir fry is a delightful combination of succulent seafood and crisp, green vegetables. Screaming with flavor and packed with nutrients, this dish offers a refreshing twist on traditional stir fries while providing essential antioxidants and anti-inflammatory compounds. Enjoy this vibrant and satisfying meal as part of your inflammation-fighting repertoire, and savor the benefits of nourishing your body with wholesome ingredients.

# Tofu and Vegetable Stir Fry with Cashew Nuts

## Ingredients:

- 1 block firm tofu, pressed and cut into cubes
- 2 cups mixed vegetables (bell peppers, broccoli, carrots, snow peas)
- 1/2 cup unsalted cashew nuts
- 2 cloves garlic, minced
- 1 tablespoon fresh ginger, grated
- 3 tablespoons low-sodium soy sauce
- 1 tablespoon hoisin sauce
- 1 tablespoon rice vinegar
- 1 teaspoon sesame oil
- 1 tablespoon olive oil
- Salt and pepper to taste
- Cooked brown rice or quinoa for serving

## Procedure:

1. Heat olive oil in a large skillet or wok over medium-high heat. Add tofu cubes and cook until golden brown on all sides, about 5-6 minutes. Remove tofu from skillet and set aside.
2. In the same skillet, add a bit more olive oil if needed. Add garlic and ginger, and cook for 1-2 minutes until fragrant.
3. Add mixed vegetables to the skillet and stir fry until crisp-tender, about 3-4 minutes.
4. Return cooked tofu to the skillet. Add soy sauce, hoisin sauce, rice vinegar, and

sesame oil. Stir well to combine and coat the ingredients evenly.

5. Cook for an additional 2-3 minutes, until the sauce has thickened slightly and everything is heated through.
6. Stir in cashew nuts and cook for another minute.
7. Serve hot over cooked brown rice or quinoa.

This sauce offers a delightful medley of flavors and textures, perfect for satisfying your cravings while supporting inflammation relief. Tofu provides a plant-based source of protein, while the colorful array of vegetables and crunchy cashew nuts add essential nutrients and antioxidants to your meal. With its savory sauce and satisfying ingredients, this stir fry is sure to become a favorite in your anti-inflammatory diet repertoire.

## Beef and Broccoli Stir Fry

**Ingredients:**
- 1 lb flank steak, thinly sliced against the grain
- 2 cups broccoli florets
- 1 red bell pepper, sliced
- 2 cloves garlic, minced
- 1 tablespoon fresh ginger, grated
- 3 tablespoons low-sodium soy sauce
- 1 tablespoon oyster sauce
- 1 tablespoon rice vinegar
- 1 teaspoon sesame oil

- 1 tablespoon olive oil
- Salt and pepper to taste
- Cooked brown rice or quinoa for serving

## Procedure:

1. Heat olive oil in a large skillet or wok over medium-high heat. Add garlic and ginger, and cook for 1-2 minutes until fragrant.
2. Add sliced beef to the skillet and cook until browned, about 2-3 minutes per side. Remove beef from skillet and set aside.
3. In the same skillet, add a bit more olive oil if needed. Add broccoli florets and sliced bell pepper, and stir fry until crisp-tender, about 3-4 minutes.
4. Return cooked beef to the skillet. Add soy sauce, oyster sauce, rice vinegar, and sesame oil. Stir well to combine and coat the ingredients evenly.
5. Cook for an additional 2-3 minutes, until the sauce has thickened slightly and everything is heated through.
6. Serve hot over cooked brown rice or quinoa.

This is a classic favorite that never fails to impress with its bold flavors and hearty ingredients. With tender slices of beef, vibrant broccoli florets, and a savory sauce infused with garlic and ginger, this dish is a surefire way to satisfy your cravings while promoting inflammation relief. Enjoy the wholesome goodness of this delicious stir fry as part of your anti-inflammatory meal plan and reap the benefits of nourishing your body with wholesome ingredients.

## Salmon and Vegetable Stir Fry

**Ingredients:**

- 1 lb salmon fillets, cut into bite-sized pieces
- 2 cups mixed vegetables (zucchini, bell peppers, carrots, snow peas)
- 2 cloves garlic, minced
- 1 tablespoon fresh ginger, grated
- 3 tablespoons low-sodium soy sauce
- 1 tablespoon honey or maple syrup
- 1 tablespoon rice vinegar
- 1 teaspoon sesame oil
- 1 tablespoon olive oil
- Salt and pepper to taste
- Cooked brown rice or quinoa for serving

**Procedure:**

1. Heat olive oil in a large skillet or wok over medium-high heat. Add garlic and ginger, and cook for 1-2 minutes until fragrant.
2. Add salmon pieces to the skillet and cook until browned on all sides and cooked through, about 3-4 minutes. Remove salmon from skillet and set aside.
3. In the same skillet, add a bit more olive oil if needed. Add mixed vegetables and stir fry until crisp-tender, about 3-4 minutes.
4. Return cooked salmon to the skillet. Add soy sauce, honey or maple syrup, rice

vinegar, and sesame oil. Stir well to combine and coat the ingredients evenly.

5.  Cook for an additional 2-3 minutes, until the sauce has thickened slightly and everything is heated through.

6.  Serve hot over cooked brown rice or quinoa.

This sauce offers a delightful combination of omega-3-rich salmon and colorful vegetables, making it a standout choice for inflammation relief. With its savory sauce and tender chunks of salmon, this dish provides a satisfying and nutritious meal that is sure to please your palate and support your overall health. Enjoy the vibrant flavors and nourishing ingredients of this delicious stir fry as part of your anti-inflammatory diet plan.

## Vegetarian Tofu and Mushroom Stir Fry

**Ingredients:**

- 1 block firm tofu, pressed and cut into cubes
- 2 cups mixed mushrooms (such as shiitake, button, and oyster), sliced
- 1 bell pepper, thinly sliced
- 1 cup snow peas, trimmed
- 2 cloves garlic, minced
- 1 tablespoon fresh ginger, grated
- 3 tablespoons low-sodium soy sauce
- 1 tablespoon hoisin sauce
- 1 tablespoon rice vinegar
- 1 teaspoon sesame oil

- 1 tablespoon olive oil
- Salt and pepper to taste
- Cooked brown rice or quinoa for serving

**Procedure:**

1. Heat olive oil in a large skillet or wok over medium-high heat. Add garlic and ginger, and cook for 1-2 minutes until fragrant.
2. Add tofu cubes to the skillet and cook until golden brown on all sides, about 5-6 minutes. Remove tofu from skillet and set aside.
3. In the same skillet, add a bit more olive oil if needed. Add mushrooms and bell pepper, and stir fry until mushrooms are golden brown and bell pepper is tender, about 4-5 minutes.
4. Add snow peas to the skillet and cook for an additional 2 minutes.
5. Return cooked tofu to the skillet. Add soy sauce, hoisin sauce, rice vinegar, and sesame oil. Stir well to combine and coat the ingredients evenly.
6. Cook for another 2-3 minutes, until the sauce has thickened slightly and everything is heated through.
7. Serve hot over cooked brown rice or quinoa.

This broth is a delightful meat-free option that doesn't skimp on flavor or nutrition. With its hearty tofu cubes, savory mushrooms, and crisp vegetables, this dish offers a satisfying and wholesome meal that is perfect for those following an anti-inflammatory diet. Packed with plant-based protein, fiber, and essential vitamins and minerals, this stir fry is sure to please your taste buds while supporting your overall health and well-being.

## Ginger Garlic Chicken Stir Fry

### Ingredients:

- 1 lb boneless, skinless chicken breast, thinly sliced
- 1 red bell pepper, sliced
- 1 yellow bell pepper, sliced
- 1 cup broccoli florets
- 2 cloves garlic, minced
- 1 tablespoon fresh ginger, grated
- 3 tablespoons low-sodium soy sauce
- 1 tablespoon honey or maple syrup
- 1 tablespoon rice vinegar
- 1 teaspoon sesame oil
- 1 tablespoon olive oil
- Salt and pepper to taste
- Cooked brown rice or quinoa for serving

### Procedure:

1. Heat olive oil in a large skillet or wok over medium-high heat. Add garlic and ginger, and cook for 1-2 minutes until fragrant.
2. Add sliced chicken breast to the skillet and cook until browned and cooked through, about 5-6 minutes. Remove chicken from skillet and set aside.

3. In the same skillet, add a bit more olive oil if needed. Add sliced bell peppers and broccoli florets, and stir fry until crisp-tender, about 3-4 minutes.
4. Return cooked chicken to the skillet. Add soy sauce, honey or maple syrup, rice vinegar, and sesame oil. Stir well to combine and coat the ingredients evenly.
5. Cook for an additional 2-3 minutes, until the sauce has thickened slightly and everything is heated through.
6. Serve hot over cooked brown rice or quinoa.

This is a flavor-packed dish that's sure to satisfy your cravings while supporting inflammation relief. With its aromatic spices, tender chicken, and vibrant vegetables, this stir fry offers a mouthwatering combination of flavors and textures that will tantalize your taste buds. Plus, with the added benefits of ginger and garlic, known for their anti-inflammatory properties, this dish is an excellent choice for those looking to promote overall health and well-being.

## Thai Basil Beef Stir Fry

**Ingredients:**
- 1 lb flank steak, thinly sliced against the grain
- 1 red bell pepper, sliced
- 1 yellow bell pepper, sliced
- 1 onion, thinly sliced

- 2 cloves garlic, minced
- 1 tablespoon fresh ginger, grated
- 3 tablespoons low-sodium soy sauce
- 1 tablespoon fish sauce
- 1 tablespoon oyster sauce
- 1 tablespoon rice vinegar
- 1 teaspoon sesame oil
- 1 tablespoon olive oil
- 1 cup fresh Thai basil leaves
- Salt and pepper to taste
- Cooked brown rice or quinoa for serving

## Procedure:

1. Heat olive oil in a large skillet or wok over medium-high heat. Add garlic and ginger, and cook for 1-2 minutes until fragrant.
2. Add sliced flank steak to the skillet and cook until browned, about 2-3 minutes per side. Remove beef from skillet and set aside.
3. In the same skillet, add a bit more olive oil if needed. Add sliced bell peppers and onion, and stir fry until peppers are tender-crisp, about 3-4 minutes.
4. Return cooked beef to the skillet. Add soy sauce, fish sauce, oyster sauce, rice vinegar, and sesame oil. Stir well to combine and coat the ingredients evenly.
5. Cook for an additional 2-3 minutes, until the sauce has thickened slightly and everything is heated through.
6. Stir in fresh Thai basil leaves and cook for another minute until wilted.

7. Serve hot over cooked brown rice or quinoa.

This offers a tantalizing fusion of flavors inspired by Thai cuisine, making it a delightful addition to your anti-inflammatory meal plan. With its tender slices of beef, colorful bell peppers, and aromatic Thai basil, this dish is sure to transport your taste buds to new heights of culinary delight. Plus, with the added benefits of ginger and garlic, this stir fry provides powerful anti-inflammatory properties that can help support your overall health and well-being.

## Spicy Tofu and Vegetable Stir Fry

**Ingredients:**
- 1 block firm tofu, pressed and cut into cubes
- 2 cups mixed vegetables (such as bell peppers, broccoli, carrots, snap peas)
- 2 cloves garlic, minced
- 1 tablespoon fresh ginger, grated
- 3 tablespoons low-sodium soy sauce
- 1 tablespoon Sriracha sauce (adjust to taste)
- 1 tablespoon rice vinegar
- 1 teaspoon sesame oil
- 1 tablespoon olive oil
- Salt and pepper to taste
- Cooked brown rice or quinoa for serving

## Procedure:

1. Heat olive oil in a large skillet or wok over medium-high heat. Add garlic and ginger, and cook for 1-2 minutes until fragrant.
2. Add tofu cubes to the skillet and cook until golden brown on all sides, about 5-6 minutes. Remove tofu from skillet and set aside.
3. In the same skillet, add a bit more olive oil if needed. Add mixed vegetables and stir fry until crisp-tender, about 3-4 minutes.
4. Return cooked tofu to the skillet. Add soy sauce, Sriracha sauce, rice vinegar, and sesame oil. Stir well to combine and coat the ingredients evenly.
5. Cook for an additional 2-3 minutes, until the sauce has thickened slightly and everything is heated through.
6. Serve hot over cooked brown rice or quinoa.

This spicy sauce is a fiery yet flavorful dish that's perfect for those who crave a little heat in their meals. With its zesty combination of tofu, mixed vegetables, and bold spices, this stir fry offers a satisfying and nutritious option for inflammation relief. Plus, with the added kick of Sriracha sauce, this dish is sure to awaken your taste buds and leave you craving more. Enjoy the vibrant flavors and nourishing ingredients of this delicious stir fry as part of your anti-inflammatory diet plan.

# Mushroom and Spinach Stir Fry

## Ingredients:

- 2 cups sliced mushrooms (such as button, cremini, or shiitake)
- 4 cups fresh spinach leaves
- 2 cloves garlic, minced
- 1 tablespoon fresh ginger, grated
- 3 tablespoons low-sodium soy sauce
- 1 tablespoon hoisin sauce
- 1 tablespoon rice vinegar
- 1 teaspoon sesame oil
- 1 tablespoon olive oil
- Salt and pepper to taste
- Cooked brown rice or quinoa for serving

## Procedure:

1. Heat olive oil in a large skillet or wok over medium-high heat. Add garlic and ginger, and cook for 1-2 minutes until fragrant.
2. Add sliced mushrooms to the skillet and cook until golden brown and tender, about 4-5 minutes.
3. Add fresh spinach leaves to the skillet and cook until wilted, about 2-3 minutes.
4. In a small bowl, whisk together soy sauce, hoisin sauce, rice vinegar, and sesame oil.
5. Pour the sauce over the mushrooms and spinach in the skillet. Stir well to combine and coat the ingredients evenly.

6. Cook for an additional 2-3 minutes, until the sauce has thickened slightly and everything is heated through.
7. Season with salt and pepper to taste.
8. Serve hot over cooked brown rice or quinoa.

This meal is a simple yet flavorful dish that celebrates the earthy flavors of mushrooms and the vibrant freshness of spinach. With its savory sauce and nutritious ingredients, this stir fry offers a satisfying and wholesome option for inflammation relief. Packed with essential vitamins, minerals, and antioxidants, this dish is sure to nourish your body and support your overall health and well-being.

## Sesame Ginger Vegetable Stir Fry

**Ingredients:**

- 2 cups mixed vegetables (such as bell peppers, carrots, snap peas, broccoli)
- 2 cloves garlic, minced
- 1 tablespoon fresh ginger, grated
- 3 tablespoons low-sodium soy sauce
- 1 tablespoon honey or maple syrup
- 1 tablespoon rice vinegar
- 1 teaspoon sesame oil
- 1 tablespoon olive oil
- 1 tablespoon sesame seeds
- Salt and pepper to taste
- Cooked brown rice or quinoa for serving

## Procedure:

1. Heat olive oil in a large skillet or wok over medium-high heat. Add garlic and ginger, and cook for 1-2 minutes until fragrant.
2. Add mixed vegetables to the skillet and stir fry until crisp-tender, about 3-4 minutes.
3. In a small bowl, whisk together soy sauce, honey or maple syrup, rice vinegar, and sesame oil.
4. Pour the sauce over the vegetables in the skillet. Stir well to combine and coat the ingredients evenly.
5. Cook for an additional 2-3 minutes, until the sauce has thickened slightly and everything is heated through.
6. Sprinkle sesame seeds over the stir fry and stir to incorporate.
7. Season with salt and pepper to taste.
8. Serve hot over cooked brown rice or quinoa.

This dressing is a delightful combination of savory and sweet flavours, with a hint of nuttiness from the sesame seeds. Packed with colourful vegetables and aromatic spices, this stir fry offers a nutritious and delicious option for inflammation relief. With its simple yet flavorful sauce, this dish is sure to please your taste buds while nourishing your body with wholesome ingredients.

# Lemon Garlic Shrimp Stir Fry

**Ingredients:**

- 1 lb large shrimp, peeled and deveined
- Zest and juice of 1 lemon
- 2 cloves garlic, minced
- 1 tablespoon fresh ginger, grated
- 3 tablespoons low-sodium soy sauce
- 1 tablespoon honey or maple syrup
- 1 tablespoon olive oil
- Salt and pepper to taste
- Cooked brown rice or quinoa for serving
- Chopped fresh parsley for garnish (optional)

**Procedure:**

1. In a small bowl, whisk together lemon zest, lemon juice, minced garlic, grated ginger, soy sauce, and honey or maple syrup.
2. Heat olive oil in a large skillet or wok over medium-high heat. Add shrimp to the skillet and cook until pink and opaque, about 2-3 minutes per side.
3. Pour the lemon garlic sauce over the shrimp in the skillet. Stir well to combine and coat the shrimp evenly.
4. Cook for an additional 1-2 minutes, until the sauce has thickened slightly and everything is heated through.
5. Season with salt and pepper to taste.
6. Serve hot over cooked brown rice or quinoa.
7. Garnish with chopped fresh parsley, if desired.

This meal is a light and refreshing dish that bursts with zesty citrus flavours and aromatic garlic. With its succulent shrimp and vibrant sauce, this stir fry offers a tantalising option for inflammation relief. Rich in protein and bursting with flavour, this dish is sure to satisfy your cravings while supporting your overall health and well-being.

## Honey Garlic Tofu Stir Fry

Ingredients:
- 1 block firm tofu, pressed and cut into cubes
- 2 cups mixed vegetables (such as bell peppers, broccoli, carrots, snap peas)
- 2 cloves garlic, minced
- 1 tablespoon fresh ginger, grated
- 3 tablespoons low-sodium soy sauce
- 2 tablespoons honey
- 1 tablespoon rice vinegar
- 1 teaspoon sesame oil
- 1 tablespoon olive oil
- Salt and pepper to taste
- Cooked brown rice or quinoa for serving

### Procedure:
1. Heat olive oil in a large skillet or wok over medium-high heat. Add garlic and ginger, and cook for 1-2 minutes until fragrant.
2. Add tofu cubes to the skillet and cook until golden brown on all sides, about 5-6

minutes. Remove tofu from skillet and set aside.

3. In the same skillet, add a bit more olive oil if needed. Add mixed vegetables and stir fry until crisp-tender, about 3-4 minutes.
4. Return cooked tofu to the skillet. In a small bowl, whisk together soy sauce, honey, and rice vinegar. Pour the sauce over the tofu and vegetables in the skillet. Stir well to combine and coat the ingredients evenly.
5. Cook for an additional 2-3 minutes, until the sauce has thickened slightly and everything is heated through.
6. Season with salt and pepper to taste.
7. Serve hot over cooked brown rice or quinoa.

This is a delightful combination of sweet and savory flavors, with a hint of tanginess from the rice vinegar. Packed with protein-rich tofu and colorful vegetables, this stir fry offers a nutritious and satisfying option for inflammation relief. With its simple yet flavorful sauce, this dish is sure to please your palate while supporting your overall health and well-being.

## Teriyaki Chicken and Vegetable Stir Fry

**Ingredients:**

- 1 lb boneless, skinless chicken breast, thinly sliced

- 2 cups mixed vegetables (such as bell peppers, broccoli, carrots, snap peas)
- 2 cloves garlic, minced
- 1 tablespoon fresh ginger, grated
- 3 tablespoons low-sodium soy sauce
- 2 tablespoons honey or maple syrup
- 1 tablespoon rice vinegar
- 1 teaspoon sesame oil
- 1 tablespoon olive oil
- 1 tablespoon cornstarch (optional, for thickening sauce)
- Salt and pepper to taste
- Cooked brown rice or quinoa for serving

## Procedure:

1. Heat olive oil in a large skillet or wok over medium-high heat. Add garlic and ginger, and cook for 1-2 minutes until fragrant.
2. Add sliced chicken breast to the skillet and cook until browned and cooked through, about 5-6 minutes. Remove chicken from skillet and set aside.
3. In the same skillet, add a bit more olive oil if needed. Add mixed vegetables and stir fry until crisp-tender, about 3-4 minutes.
4. In a small bowl, whisk together soy sauce, honey or maple syrup, rice vinegar, and sesame oil. If desired, whisk in cornstarch to thicken the sauce.
5. Return cooked chicken to the skillet. Pour the sauce over the chicken and vegetables.

Stir well to combine and coat the ingredients evenly.

6. Cook for an additional 2-3 minutes, until the sauce has thickened slightly and everything is heated through.
7. Season with salt and pepper to taste.
8. Serve hot over cooked brown rice or quinoa.

This garnish is a classic favourite that's sure to please your taste buds while supporting inflammation relief. With its tender chicken, crisp vegetables, and flavorful teriyaki sauce, this stir fry offers a satisfying and nutritious option for a wholesome meal. Packed with essential nutrients and bursting with flavor, this dish is perfect for enjoying with your favorite grain such as brown rice or quinoa.

## Pineapple Shrimp Stir Fry

**Ingredients:**
- 1 lb large shrimp, peeled and deveined
- 2 cups pineapple chunks (fresh or canned)
- 1 bell pepper, sliced
- 1 onion, thinly sliced
- 2 cloves garlic, minced
- 1 tablespoon fresh ginger, grated
- 3 tablespoons low-sodium soy sauce
- 2 tablespoons honey or maple syrup
- 1 tablespoon rice vinegar
- 1 teaspoon sesame oil
- 1 tablespoon olive oil

- Salt and pepper to taste
- Cooked brown rice or quinoa for serving

## Procedure:

1. Heat olive oil in a large skillet or wok over medium-high heat. Add garlic and ginger, and cook for 1-2 minutes until fragrant.
2. Add shrimp to the skillet and cook until pink and opaque, about 2-3 minutes per side. Remove shrimp from skillet and set aside.
3. In the same skillet, add a bit more olive oil if needed. Add bell pepper and onion, and stir fry until peppers are tender-crisp, about 3-4 minutes.
4. Add pineapple chunks to the skillet and cook for an additional 1-2 minutes.
5. Return cooked shrimp to the skillet. In a small bowl, whisk together soy sauce, honey or maple syrup, and rice vinegar. Pour the sauce over the shrimp and vegetables in the skillet. Stir well to combine and coat the ingredients evenly.
6. Cook for another 2-3 minutes, until the sauce has thickened slightly and everything is heated through.
7. Season with salt and pepper to taste.
8. Serve hot over cooked brown rice or quinoa.

This side dish is a tropical delight that combines the sweet and tangy flavors of pineapple with succulent shrimp and crisp vegetables. With its vibrant colors and refreshing taste, this stir fry offers a delicious and nutritious option for inflammation relief. Packed with protein, vitamins, and minerals, this dish is sure to satisfy your cravings while nourishing your body with wholesome ingredients.

## Conclusion

In conclusion, stir fry dishes are not only delicious and versatile but also offer numerous benefits for individuals seeking to alleviate inflammation and improve their overall health. By incorporating a variety of colorful vegetables, lean proteins, and flavorful sauces, stir fries provide a convenient and satisfying way to enjoy nutrient-rich meals while supporting inflammation relief.

Throughout this chapter, we've explored 15 diverse stir fry recipes, each designed to tantalize your taste buds and promote inflammation relief. From shrimp and tofu to chicken and beef, these stir fry dishes showcase the endless possibilities for creating wholesome and flavorful meals that nourish both body and soul.

Whether you're a novice in the kitchen or a seasoned chef, these recipes offer something for everyone to enjoy. With their simple ingredients, easy preparation, and delicious results, stir fries are an excellent addition to any anti-inflammatory diet.

So why wait? Start experimenting with these flavorful stir fry recipes today and embark on a culinary journey that not only delights your palate but also supports your journey towards improved health and well-being. Stay tuned for more inspiring recipes and helpful tips to enhance your anti-inflammatory lifestyle.

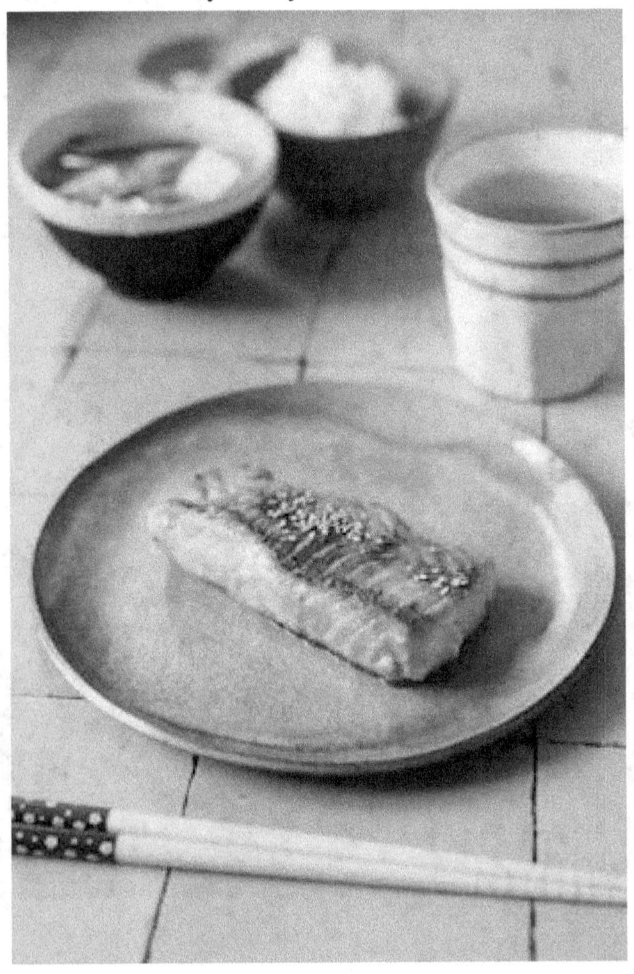

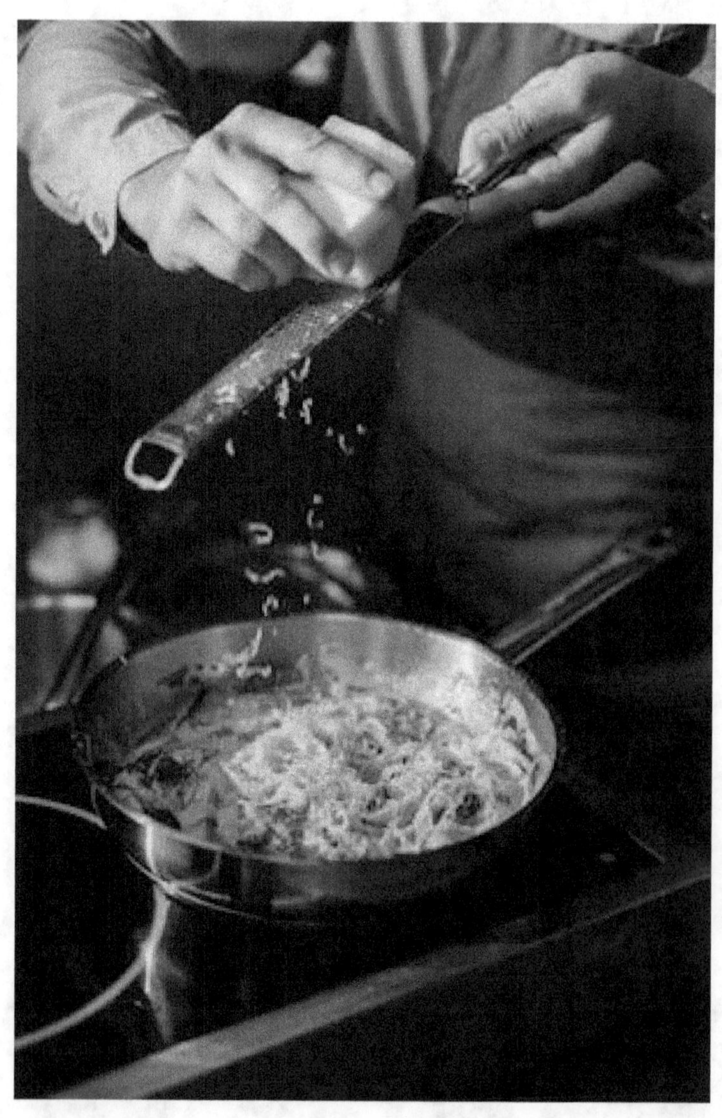

# CHAPTER NINE

## The Anti-inflammatory Lifestyle

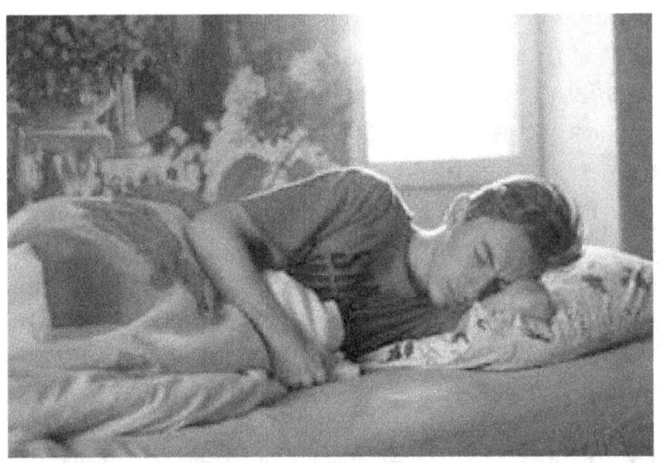

Living an anti-inflammatory lifestyle is crucial for managing inflammation and promoting overall health and well-being. In this chapter, we'll delve deep into practical strategies and techniques to incorporate into your daily routine to reduce inflammation effectively.

## Stress and Inflammation

Chronic stress is a significant contributor to inflammation in the body. When you experience stress, your body releases cortisol and other stress hormones, which can trigger inflammation. Therefore, it's essential to implement stress reduction techniques to mitigate its impact. Here are some effective strategies:

## Mindfulness Meditation

Mindfulness meditation involves focusing your attention on the present moment without judgment. Research has shown that regular meditation can reduce stress levels and lower inflammation markers in the body. Set aside a few minutes each day to practice mindfulness meditation, even if it's just for a short period. Simply sit quietly, close your eyes, and focus on your breath, observing any thoughts or sensations that arise without judgment.

## Deep Breathing Exercises

Deep breathing exercises can help activate the body's relaxation response, reducing cortisol levels and promoting a sense of calmness. Practice deep breathing by inhaling deeply through your nose, filling your lungs with air, and exhaling slowly through your mouth. Repeat this process several times, focusing on the sensation of your breath as it enters and leaves your body.

## Regular Exercise

Engaging in regular physical activity is not only beneficial for your physical health but also for managing stress and reducing inflammation. Aim for at least 30 minutes of moderate exercise most days of the week. Activities like brisk walking, cycling, swimming, or yoga can help lower stress levels and promote overall well-being.

## Practice Gratitude

Take a few moments each day to reflect on the things you're grateful for. Keeping a gratitude journal or simply mentally noting three things you're thankful for can help shift your focus away from stressors and cultivate a more positive mindset.

## Engage in Relaxation Techniques

Explore different relaxation techniques such as progressive muscle relaxation, guided imagery, or autogenic training. These practices can help activate the body's relaxation response and reduce stress levels.

## Connect with Nature

Spending time outdoors and connecting with nature can have a calming effect on the mind and body. Take a walk in the park, go for a hike, or simply sit outside and enjoy the sights and sounds of nature to help alleviate stress.

## Set Boundaries

Learn to say no to activities or commitments that add unnecessary stress to your life. Setting boundaries and prioritizing your own well-being is essential for managing stress and maintaining balance in your life.

Implementing these stress-alleviating techniques can help you effectively manage stress and cultivate a greater sense of calm and well-being in your life.

# Sleep and Inflammation

Quality sleep is essential for maintaining a healthy inflammatory response in the body. During sleep, your body repairs and rejuvenates itself, including the immune system. Lack of sleep can disrupt this process and increase inflammation levels. Here's how you can prioritize sleep for inflammation management:

## Establish a Consistent Sleep Schedule

Try to go to bed and wake up at the same time every day, even on weekends. Consistency is key to regulating your body's internal clock and promoting restful sleep. Create a relaxing bedtime routine to signal to your body that it's time to wind down, such as taking a warm bath, reading a book, or practicing relaxation techniques.

## Create a Sleep-friendly Environment

Make sure your bedroom is conducive to sleep by keeping it cool, dark, and quiet. Invest in a comfortable mattress and pillows that support your sleep posture. Limit exposure to electronic devices like smartphones and computers before bedtime, as the blue light emitted from screens can disrupt your sleep-wake cycle.

## Prioritize Sleep Hygiene

Practice good sleep hygiene habits to improve the quality of your sleep. Avoid consuming caffeine or alcohol close to bedtime, as they can interfere with your sleep patterns. Additionally, limit daytime naps to avoid disrupting your nighttime sleep. If you're having trouble sleeping, consider consulting with a healthcare professional for further guidance.

## Limit Exposure to Screens Before Bed

The blue light emitted by electronic devices like smartphones, tablets, and computers can interfere with your body's production of melatonin, a hormone that regulates sleep-wake cycles. Aim to limit screen time at least an hour before bedtime to promote better sleep quality.

# Incorporating Physical Exercise into Your Routine

Regular physical activity is essential for reducing inflammation and promoting overall health. Exercise helps improve circulation, boost mood, and support immune function. Here's how you can incorporate exercise into your daily routine:

## Choose Activities You Enjoy

Find activities that you enjoy and are more likely to stick with long-term. Whether it's walking, jogging, dancing, or playing a sport, the key is to stay active and make it a habit.

## Mix It Up

Include a variety of activities in your exercise routine to target different muscle groups and prevent boredom. Incorporate both aerobic exercise, such as walking or cycling, and strength training exercises, like lifting weights or doing bodyweight exercises, for a well-rounded fitness regimen.

## Set Realistic Goals

Set achievable fitness goals that align with your abilities and schedule. Start small and gradually increase the intensity and duration of your workouts as your fitness level improves. Remember that consistency is more important than intensity, so aim for regular exercise rather than occasional intense workouts.

# Conclusion

Living an anti-inflammatory lifestyle requires a holistic approach that addresses stress, sleep, and physical activity. By implementing stress reduction techniques, prioritizing adequate sleep, and incorporating regular exercise into your routine, you can effectively manage inflammation and improve your overall health and well-being. In the next section, we'll explore the role of nutrition in combating inflammation and provide practical tips for incorporating anti-inflammatory foods into your diet. Stay tuned for more insights on living your best, inflammation-free life!

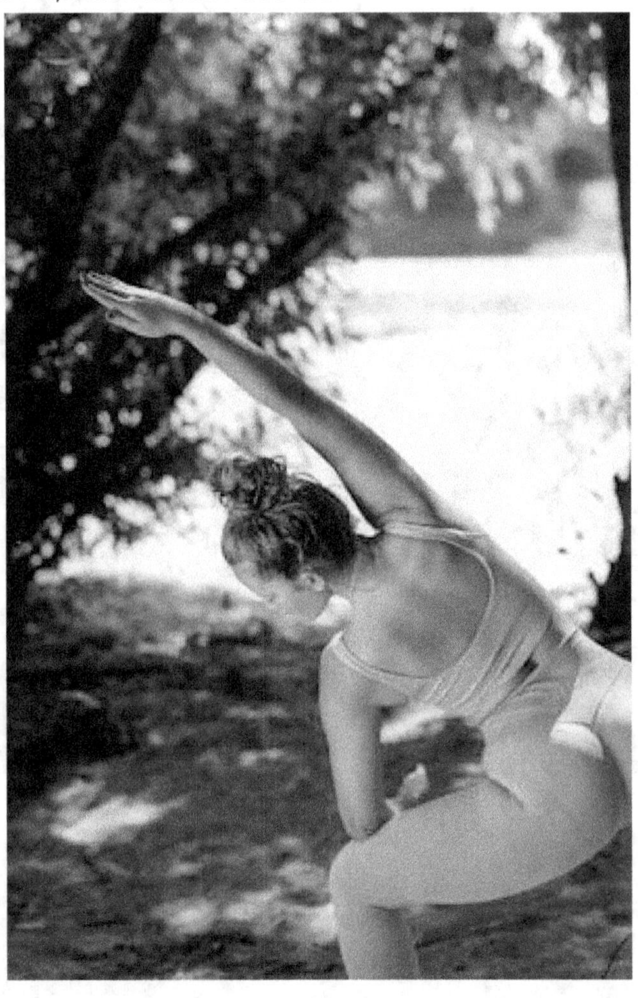

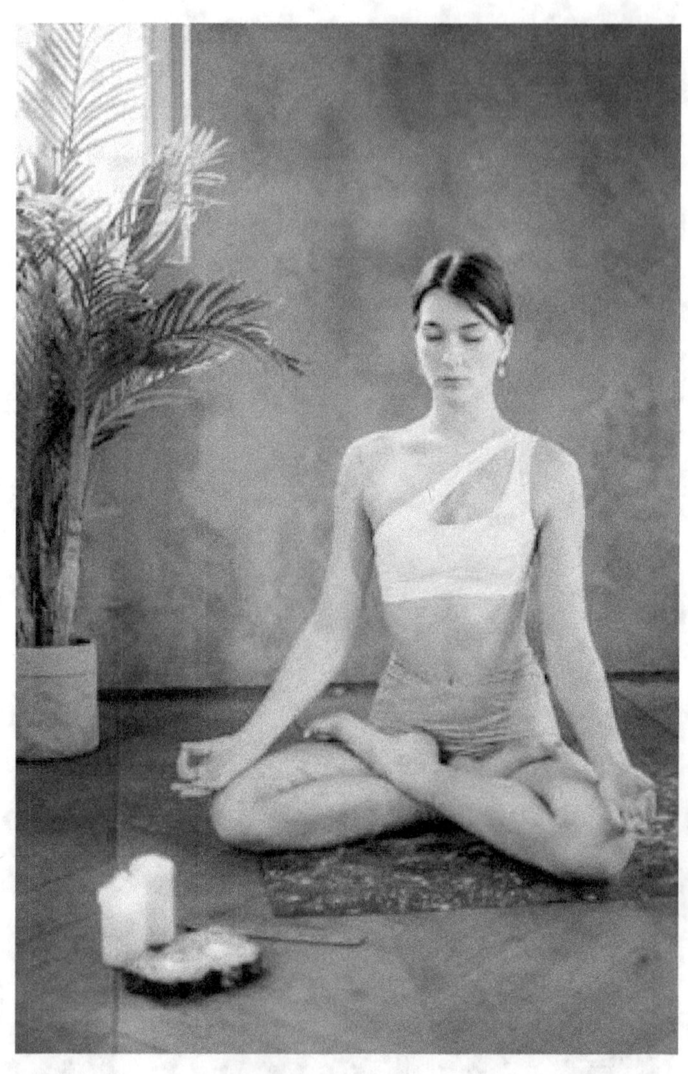

# CHAPTER TEN

## Author's Concluding Note

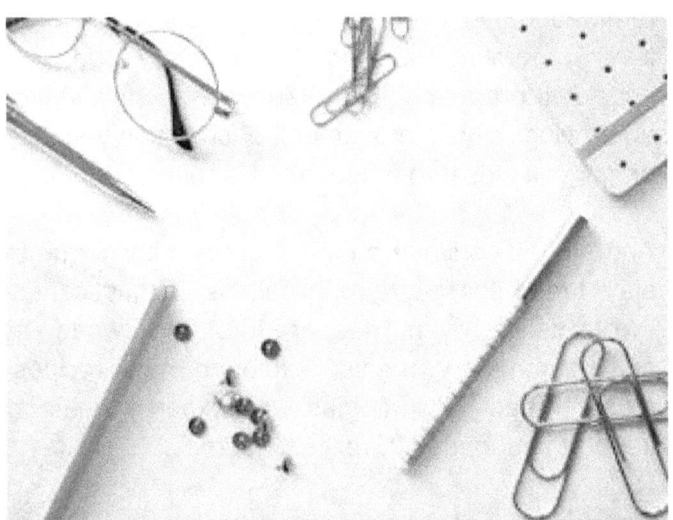

As we come to the end of this journey together, I want to express my gratitude for joining me on this exploration of the anti-inflammatory meal plans. Throughout this book, we've delved deep into the intricacies of inflammation, discovering its impact on our health and well-being. We've explored kitchen tips and culinary delights, with over 70 recipes designed to nourish your body and soothe inflammation from within.

But our journey doesn't end here. In fact, it's just the beginning. As we've uncovered the power of anti-inflammatory living, there's still so much more to explore and discover. The anti-inflammatory lifestyle is not just a one-time commitment; it's a lifelong journey towards optimal health and vitality.

As you embark on your own path towards wellness, remember that every small step counts. Whether it's incorporating more anti-inflammatory foods into your diet, practicing stress-reduction techniques, or embracing mindful movement, each action you take brings you closer to a healthier, happier you.

And as you continue on this journey, I invite you to stay tuned for future publications in this series. We'll delve even deeper into the world of anti-inflammatory meals, exploring new recipes, research-backed strategies, and expert insights to support your ongoing wellness journey.

Thank you once again for choosing to prioritize your health and well-being. Here's to a future filled with vitality, joy, and abundant health.

With warm regards,
Abel Moore

www.ingramcontent.com/pod-product-compliance
Lightning Source LLC
Chambersburg PA
CBHW061044250726
48653CB00001B/238